MCQs in De
with Explc
PG Dental Entra

MCQs in Dental Materials with Explanations for PG Dental Entrance Examinations

Also for BDS & MDS Professional Examinations

Satish Chandra

Best Teacher Awardee
Ex-Member, Dental Council of India
Ex-Director and Professor
Sardar Patel Institute of Dental and Medical Sciences, Lucknow
Ex-Professor and Head of the Department and Dean
Dental Faculty, UP KG University of Dental Sciences (Formerly, KG Medical
College, CSM Medical University and KG Medical University, Lucknow)
Ex-Professor, Dean, Head and Principal
DJ College of Dental Sciences and Research, Modinagar, UP
Ex-Professor, Dean, Head and Principal, Institute of Dental Sciences, Bareilly
Ex-Principal, Professor and Head of the Department, Awadh Institute of Dental
Sciences, Lucknow
Paper Setter and Examiner of BDS, MDS and PGME
Examinations in Many Universities
Ex-Member, Dental Council of India

Shaleen Chandra

Professor and Head of the Dept., Saraswati Dental College and Hospital,
233 Tiwariganj, Faizabad Road, Juggour, Lucknow
Ex-Professor and Head of the Dept., Sardar Patel Institute of Dental
and Medical Sciences, Lucknow
Ex-Assistant Professor, Rama Dental College and Hospital
and Research Centre, Kanpur
Ex-Lecturer, UP KG University of Dental Sciences (Formerly, KG Medical College,
CSM Medical University and KG Medical University), Lucknow
Ex-Lecturer, Buddha Institute of Dental Sciences, Kankar Bagh, Patna
Paper Setter and Examiner of BDS, MDS and PGME
Examinations in Many Universities

Girish Chandra

Rajendra Nagar Dental Clinic, Lucknow

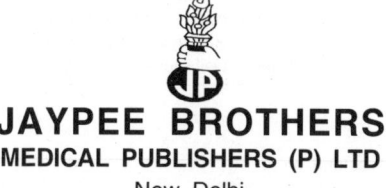

JAYPEE BROTHERS
MEDICAL PUBLISHERS (P) LTD
New Delhi

Published by

Jitendar P Vij

Jaypee Brothers Medical Publishers (P) Ltd

B-3 EMCA House, 23/23B Ansari Road, Daryaganj,
New Delhi 110 002, India Phones: +91-11-23272143, +91-11-23272703,
+91-11-23282021, +91-11-23245672, Rel: 32558559
Fax: +91-11-23276490, +91-11-23245683
e-mail: jaypee@jaypeebrothers.com
Visit our website: www.jaypeebrothers.com

Branches

- 2/B, Akruti Society, Jodhpur Gam Road Satellite
  Ahmedabad 380015, Phones: +91-079-26926233, Rel: +91-079-32988717,
  Fax: +91-079-26927094 e-mail: jpamdvd@rediffmail.com

- 202 Batavia Chambers, 8 Kumara Krupa Road, Kumara Park East
  Bangalore 560 001, Phones: +91-80-22285971, +91-80-22382956,
  Rel: +91-80-32714073 Fax: +91-80-22281761 e-mail: jaypeemedpubbgl@eth.net

- 282 IIIrd Floor, Khaleel Shirazi Estate, Fountain Plaza Pantheon Road,
  Chennai 600 008, Phones: +91-44-28193265, +91-44 28194897,
  Rel: +91-44-32972089, Fax: +91-44-28193231, e-mail: jpchen@eth.net

- 4-2-1067/1-3, Ist Floor, Balaji Building, Ramkote Cross Road
  Hyderabad 500 095, Phones: +91-40-66610020, +91-40-24758498,
  Rel: +91-40-32940929, Fax: +91-40-24758499, e-mail: jpmedpub@rediffmail.com

- 1-A Indian Mirror Street, Wellington Square,
  Kolkata 700 013, Phones: +91-33-22451926, +91-33-22276404,
  +91-33-22276415, Rel: +91-33-32901926, Fax: +91-33-22456075,
  e-mail: jpbcal@dataone.in

- 106 Amit Industrial Estate, 61 Dr SS Rao Road, Near MGM Hospital, Parel,
  Mumbai 400 012, Phones: +91-22-24124863, +91-22-24104532,
  Rel: +91-22-32926896, Fax: +91-22-24160828,
  e-mail: jpmedpub@bom7.vsnl.net.in

- "KAMALPUSHPA" 38, Reshimbag Opp Mohota Science College, Umred Road,
  Nagpur 440 009 (MS) Phone: Rel: 3245220, Fax: 0712-2704275
  e-mail: jaypeenagpur@dataone.in

MCQs in Dental Materials

© 2006, Satish Chandra, Shaleen Chandra, Girish Chandra

This book has been published in good faith that the material provided by authors is original. Every effort is made to ensure accuracy of material, but the publisher, printer and authors will not be held responsible for any inadvertent error(s). In case of any dispute, all legal matters are to be settled under Delhi jurisdiction only.

First Edition: **2006**

ISBN 81-8061-857-9

Typeset at JPBMP typesetting unit

Printed in India

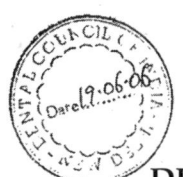 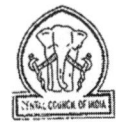 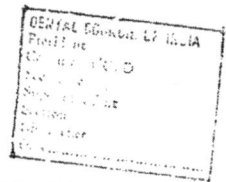

भारतीय दन्त परिषद

DENTAL COUNCIL OF INDIA
(CONSTITUTED UNDER THE DENTISTS ACT 1948)
Aiwan-E-Galib Marg, Kotla Road, New Delhi-110 002

DR. ANIL KOHLI
MDS (Lko), DNBE (USA)
President   DNO-4379
Awardee:
- Padmashri
- Padmabhushan
- Dr. B.C. Roy National Award

Telephone : 23220204 Direct
                  23238542, 23236740
               : 0091 - 11 - 23231252
                  0091 - 11 - 23220204
E- mail   : dciindia@hotmail.com
Website : http://www.dciindia.org

FOREWORD

The progressive concept is changing very fast from subjective to objective. In many universities a part of the professional examination question papers contain objective type questions.

All the competitions contain only Multiple Choice Questions (MCQs). In MCQ type objective question papers, questions from the full course can be covered, while only in subjective type question papers, it is not possible to cover the complete course of the subject, because out of an average of about 50 topics in a subject only 6 questions on 6 topics can be asked. When the question papers are of subjective type, students do only the superficial selective reading and lack the complete and deeper knowledge of the subject. With MCQ type of question papers the chances of leakage of the question papers are also very much reduced as they cover complete course of the subject and the students have to read complete course.

This book provides excellent and comprehensive coverage, covering all the aspects of the subject with unique and to the point explanations, which are in simple and easy language. This book is of great value to the students preparing for BDS and MDS and various competitive examinations.

Dr Anil Kohli
President
Dental Council of India

Preface

This book has been written keeping professional and PG Dental Entrance Examinations in mind. Answers have been given with the explanations. It is based on the experience of many toppers regarding flying success in the examinations. This book will guide in preparations for examination. The questions in this book have been compiled after analyzing many question papers of previous years.

The secret of success in competitive examination lies in proper guidance and hard work. This book simplifies your preparation by making you work more efficiently. For the sake of convenience the MCQs have been divided subjectwise, one book on each major subject. Some allied subjects have been joined together. All the books on MCQs will be true friends and a great asset for the candidates of dental professional examinations, the postgraduate dental entrance examinations and interview and also for practitioners.

The trend is very fast changing toward MCQs. These books will also be very useful for the students of graduate and postgraduate courses, as these contain questions, which are likely to be asked in periodical assessments during graduate and postgraduate courses and in final examinations.

For the preparation for examinations the aim of these books is to encourage the readers to detect areas of weakness in understanding the subject matter so that they may again study the textbooks for better and comprehensive review of the subject.

Every effort has been made to update all the books. All the books will be very useful for all the students and will prepare them to face any examination with full confidence.

Satish Chandra
Shaleen Chandra
Girish Chandra

Preface

Tips for Success

1. Start your preparations at least one year in advance. Give six months for initial preparation (Reading textbooks and solving MCQs), 4 months for final preparation (Solving MCQs from books) and last two months for revision of MCQs.

2. Procure all study materials and finish subject by subject.

3. Plan your study hours.

4. Consult your seniors who have passed the examinations with a good score. Follow their advice but not blindly.

5. Read the textbook of the subjects thoroughly from the beginning to the end. Do not do selective reading except only in revision.

6. Be organized in your study.

7. Aim for the top because you will invariably fall short.

8. Practice self-assessment tests and solve model test papers to know which chapters require revision and to get a feel of examination conditions.

9. Understand each chapter of each subject and attempt connected MCQs before proceeding to the next chapter. If you correctly answer less than 90% of MCQs, repeat the chapter.

10. Practise, practise and practise MCQs again and again with reasoning.

11. Time yourself while solving model test papers and examination question papers.

12. Relax and be tension-free while attempting questions in the examination.

13. Read the questions carefully to understand them, think and then answer.

Information and Suggestions

Remember
- You can do it. Always try for the top slots because if you aim for the sky, you would at least reach the hilltop.
- You can do it and have to do it.

Tentative dates of various entrance exams			Approximate No. of seats available
All India PG	-	Jan	130
AIIMS	-	Jan/June	4
BHU	-	Jan to March	2
PGI Chandigarh	-	June/Nov	4
MAHE	-	May	50
Various state/ College/ Universities entrances	-	Jan to Dec	1000

The following is the approximate percentage of MCQs appeared in the various postgraduate entrance examinations in previous years.

Subject	No. of MCQs %age	Weeks required for revision	
		Textbooks	MCQs books
1. Purely Preclinical	3	1	1
2. Applied Preclinical	8	2	2
3. Oral and Dental Pathology and Oral Medicine	25	5	5
4. Oral and Maxillofacial Surgery	9	2	2
5. Periodontics	5	1	1
6. Prosthodontics and Applied Dental Material	14	3	3
7. Conservative Dentistry	8	2	2
8. Orthodontics	8	2	2
9. Dental Radiology	3	2	2
10. Endodontics	5	2	2
11. Community Dentistry	2	1	1

Contd...

Contd...

Subject	No. of MCQs %age	Weeks required for revision	
		Textbooks	MCQs books
12. Gen. Medicine and Surgery	5	1	1
13. Pedodontics and Preventive Dentistry	5	1	1
Total	100	25	25

1. Only hard labor and vast knowledge are not enough but mastering the technique of taking MCQs examination is equally important.
2. First, clear the basic fundamentals to have wider and better understanding of the subject. You must read the textbooks as much as possible.
3. Do not attempt the questions that you are not sure of. Negative marks due to guesswork always take you down in the merit list. Even 1 mark can change your merit tremendously.
4. It is better to leave a question rather than to attempt it wrongly.
5. Research in psychology has concluded that most of us mark the right choice first and due to second thoughts mark a wrong choice.
6. The entrance examinations are to test the basic fundamental knowledge of the subject. Mostly the choices are straight forward and not to trick you. Answer each question from general principles rather than from exceptions.
7. Appear in all the entrance examinations in which you are eligible. You never know when luck may favor you.

Contents

Contents

1 General Properties of Dental Materials

1. **Diffusion can vary with:**
   A. Temperature
   B. Atom size
   C. Interatomic bonding
   D. All of the above

2. **For proper adhesion, the distance between the surface molecules should not be greater than:**
   A. 0.007 μm
   B. 0.0007 μm
   C. 0.07 μm
   D. 0.7 μm

3. **Contact angle formed by water on a soapy surface is:**
   A. High contact angle
   B. Medium contact angle
   C. Low contact angle
   D. None of the above

4. **Amount of energy absorbed by a structure when it is stressed not to exceed its proportional limit is:**
   A. Modulus of elasticity
   B. Flexibility
   C. Resilience
   D. Toughness

5. **Macrohardness test is /are:**
   A. Vickers test
   B. Rockwell test
   C. Brinell test
   D. Both B and C

6. **Microhardness test/s is/are:**
   A. Knoop hardness test
   B. Vickers hardness test
   C. Rockwell hardness test
   D. Both A and B

7. **Which of the following tests is used for dental casting golds?**
   A. Vickers test
   B. Knoop hardness test
   C. Rockwell test
   D. None of the above

8. **Hardness of rubber and plastics is measured from:**
   A. Knoop hardness test
   B. Rockwell test
   C. Shore and Barcol tests
   D. Brinell test

9. If a material's viscosity decreases with increase in shear rate, it is said to exhibit:
   A. Newtonian behaviour
   B. Pseudoplastic behaviour
   C. Thixotropic behaviour
   D. Dilatant behaviour

10. Liquids that show higher viscosity as shear rate increases are known as:
    A. Pseudoplastic   B. Dilatant
    C. Thixotropic   D. Newtonian

11. Degree of saturation of a particular hue is known as:
    A. Color   B. Value
    C. Chroma   D. None of the above

12. Wavelength of ultraviolet rays is:
    A. 100 to 200 nm   B. 200 to 300 nm
    C. 300 to 400 nm   D. 400 to 500 nm

13. Time dependent flow is known as:
    A. Viscosity   B. Resilience
    C. Creep   D. Toughness

14. Hardness of the materials is influenced by all of the following *except*:
    A. Strength   B. Proportional limit
    C. Ductility   D. None of the above

15. Toughness is dependent on:
    A. Ductility   B. Flexibility
    C. Elastic modulus D. All of the above

16. Ability of the materials to withstand rupture under compression is known as:
    A. Ductility   B. Hardness
    C. Malleability   D. None of the above

17. What is the effect of increase in temperature on ductility?
    A. Decrease in ductility   B. Increase in ductility
    C. Remains same   D. None of the above

18. Energy required to fracture a material is known as:
    A. Resilience   B. Malleability
    C. Toughness   D. Ductility

19. Phenomenon of static fatigue is exhibited by:
    A. Gold alloy   **B.** Ceramic material
    C. Amalgam   **D.** Composite

20. Transverse strength is used to test:
    A. Denture base resins   **B.** Long span bridges
    C. Both of the above   **D.** None of the above

21. Which of the following is used to study the interface between two materials?
    A. Flexure strength   **B.** Transverse strength
    C. Tensile strength   **D.** Shear strength

Answers

1.D. At any temperature above absolute zero, the atoms of a solid possess some amount of kinetic energy. Higher the temperature, greater the rate of diffusion. Smaller the atom size, greater the diffusion rate. Greater the interatomic bonding, lesser the rate of diffusion.

2.B. The attraction becomes negligible when the surface molecules of attracting surfaces are separated by distances greater than 0.0007 µm. (0.7 nm).

3.C. Low contact angle formed between water and a soapy surface allows water to completely wet the surface therefore water can be used to wash a soapy surface.

4.C. Resilience is the energy that is absorbed by any substance when work is done over it which brings about elastic deformation.

5.D. Brinell and Rockwell hardness tests employ loads greater than 9.8N and measure hardness over much larger areas.

6.D. Knoop and Vickers hardness tests use loads less than 9.8N and measure hardness in small regions of very thin objects. The indentations are small and less than 19 µm in depth.

7.A. In Vickers hardness test a diamond in the shape of a square-based pyramid is used. The Vickers test is employed in the American Dental Association Specification for dental casting gold. It has also been used for measuring the hardness of tooth structure.

8.C. Shore and Barcol hardness tests are sometimes employed for assessing the hardness of dental materials, particularly rubbers and plastics. The hardness number is based upon the depth of penetration of the indenter point into the material.

9.B. In pseudoplastic materials, as the amount of shear stress is increased, rate of shear strain increases and viscosity decreases until it reaches a nearly constant value.

10.B. This behaviour is opposite to that of pseudoplastic behaviour. Such liquids become more rigid as the rate of deformation increases.

11.C. Higher the chroma, more intense is the color. It is dependent on hue and value.

12.C. UV-A spectrum ranges between 320 and 400 nm and UV-B spectrum ranges between 290 and 320 nm. UV-C spectrum have wavelength below 290 nm and is completely absorbed by the ozone layer.

13.C. If a metal is held at a temperature near its melting point and is subjected to constant applied stress, the resulting strain increases as a function of time.

14.D. Strength, proportional limit and ductility influence the hardness of a material.

15.A. Toughness increases with increase in ductility. (Ductility is the total plastic strain).

16.C. Malleability is not as dependent on strength as is ductility. Most malleable and ductile pure metal is gold and silver the second.

17.A. The ability of a material to withstand permanent deformation under a tensile load without rupture is called ductility. It depends upon tensile strength. In general, ductility, decreases with increase in temperature.

18.C. Toughness is the measure of resistance to fracture. Greater the amount of energy required to fracture a material, tougher is the material.

19.B. In case of ceramics, constant tensile stress along with an aqueous corrosive medium leads to degradation of the ceramic.

20.C. Transverse strength is also known as flexure strength or modulus of rupture.

21.D. A stress that tends to resist a twisting motion or sliding of one portion of a body over another is known as a shear stress which results from the forces that act parallel to the surface of the objects.

2 Biocompatibility of Dental Materials

1. If the materials injure the pulp then which of the following properties of dental materials is/are unimportant?
   A. Strength
   B. Resistance to corrosion
   C. Both of the above
   D. None of the above

2. Which of the following tests is not included in initial or primary test?
   A. Genetotoxicity test
   B. Cytotoxicity assays
   C. Mutagenesis assays
   D. None of the above

3. Microleakage results in:
   A. Secondary caries   B. Discoloration
   C. Sensitivity   D. All of the above

4. Which of the following tests is not included in intermediate or secondary test for biocompatibility of dental materials?
   A. Systemic toxicity test
   B. Inhalation toxicity test
   C. Mucous membrane irritation test
   D. None of the above

5. Toxicity tests are classified into all of the following *except*:
   A. Screening test   B. Usage test
   C. Human trials   D. None of the above

6. All of the following materials are used for fabrication of implant *except*:
   A. Metals   B. Alloys
   C. Ceramics   D. None of the above

7. Which of the followings is not present in vitallium?
   A. Nickel   B. Cobalt
   C. Chromium   D. Molybdenum

Answers

1.C. Conduciveness to the pulp is the primary requisite of a restorative material.

2.D. Genetotoxicity test, cytotoxicity assays and mutagenesis assays are all primary tests for testing biocompatibility of dental materials.

3.D. Microleakage along tooth-restoration interface leads to percolation of bacteria below the restoration, which cause sensitivity, secondary caries, and discoloration of the tooth.

4.D. Systemic toxicity, inhalation toxicity and mucous membrane irritation caused by a dental material are measured in the secondary tests.

5.D. Screening test, usage test and human trials all are tests for evaluating the toxicity of dental materials.

6.D. Fabrication of implants can be done from metal, ceramics or alloys.

7.A. Vitallium is the name commonly associated with the alloys used in dental and medical (implant) applications. These alloys mainly contain 60% cobalt and 25% chromium.

1. Type III gypsum product is also known as:
   A. Dental plaster
   B. Medium strength stone
   C. High strength stone
   D. Dental stone, high strength, high expansion

2. Orthorhombic anhydrite is formed at temperature between:
   A. 110–130° C
   B. 130–200° C
   C. 200–1000° C
   D. 1000–1350° C

3. Type IV dental stone is also known as:
   A. Dental plaster high strength
   B. Dental stone
   C. Improved stone
   D. Dental stone, high strength, high expansion

4. Recommended W:P ratio for improved stone (type IV) is:
   A. 0.45:0.50   B. 0.28:0.30
   C. 0.22:0.24   D. 0.18:0.22

5. To manufacture improved stone which of the following is used?
   A. Calcium sulfate   B. Calcium chloride
   C. Potassium sulfate   D. Potassium chloride

6. How many times hemihydrate is more soluble than dihydrate?
   A. Two times   B. Three times
   C. Four times   D. None of the above

7. Water requirement of a product is affected by:
   A. Compactness and shape of crystals
   B. Small amount of surface active materials
   C. Particle size distribution
   D. All of the above

8. Recommended W:P ratio for dental stone is:
   - A. 0.18:0.22
   - B. 0.28:0.30
   - C. 0.50:0.75
   - D. 0.22:0.24

9. Maximum setting expansion at 2 hours of high strength dental stone is:
   - A. 0.10%
   - B. 0.15%
   - C. 0.20%
   - D. 0.30%

10. Compressive strength at 1 hour of high strength and high expansion dental stone is:
   - A. 1300 psi
   - B. 3000 psi
   - C. 5000 psi
   - D. 7000 psi

11. Diameter of the Vicat needle is:
   - A. 1.0 mm
   - B. 1.5 mm
   - C. 2.0 mm
   - D. 2.5 mm

12. Weight of large Gillmore needle is:
   - A. 0.5 lb
   - B. 0.25 lb
   - C. 1 lb
   - D. 2 lb

13. Which of the following factors affect/s setting time of plaster of Paris?
   - A. Mixing and spatulation
   - B. Manufacturing process
   - C. Temperature
   - D. All of the above

14. Plaster will set faster in all of the following conditions *except*:
   - A. If excess gypsum is left in the final product
   - B. If soluble anhydrate is less
   - C. If natural anhydrate is in excess
   - D. If particle size is fine

15. Upto which concentration sodium sulfate acts as accelerator?
   - A. 2%
   - B. 3.4%
   - C. 3.0%
   - D. 2.8%

16. Which of the following is/are an accelerator?
   - A. Sodium chloride
   - B. Potassium sulfate
   - C. Sodium sulfate
   - D. All of the above

17. Which of the followings is not a retarder?
    A. Acetates   B. Citrates
    C. Ferric sulfate   D. None of the above

18. Most effective retarder for setting of gypsum is:
    A. Acetates   B. Borax
    C. Sodium chloride   D. Sodium sulfate

19. Terra alba acts as:
    A. Accelerator for setting of gypsum
    B. Retarder for setting of gypsum
    C. Both of the above
    D. None of the above

20. Normal setting expansion of gypsum is:
    A. 0.06%–0.5%   B. 0.005–0.05%
    C. 0.01–0.1%   D. 0.1–1.0%

21. All of the following increases setting expansion of gypsum
    except:
    A. Increased spatulation
    B. Decreased W:P ratio
    C. Sodium chloride
    D. Ground gypsum

22. Four percent solution of potassium sulfate reduces the setting
    expansion of gypsum to:
    A. 0.5%   B. 0.05%
    C. 0.06%   D. 0.01%

23. Wet strength for improved dental stone is:
    A. 9 MPa   B. 25 MPa
    C. 35 MPa   D. 40 MPa

24. Which of the following factors reduce the strength of dental
    stone?
    A. Addition of accelerators
    B. Addition of retarders
    C. Both of the above
    D. None of the above

25. At least how much percentage of one hour strength is necessary
    for the cast to be used?
    A. 50%   B. 80%
    C. 90%   D. 95%

26. In which of the following potato starch is present?
    A. Impression plaster   B. Model plaster
    C. Soluble plaster   D. Dental stone

27. Rochelle salt is:
    A. Potassium chloride
    B. Potassium sodium tartarate
    C. Sodium citrate
    D. Sodium tetraborate decahydrate

28. Setting expansion of dental stone is:
    A. 0.01%-0.1%   B. 0.06%-0.12%
    C. 0.5%-0.1%   D. 0.05-0.5%

29. Which of the following types of gypsum products is also known as die stone?
    A. Type I   B. Type II
    C. Type III   D. Type IV

30. Dental stone consists of all of the following *except*:
    A. Alphahemihydrate
    B. K_2SO_4 as an accelerator
    C. Borax as a retarder
    D. None of the above

31. Setting expansion of type V dental stone is:
    A. 0.10%   B. 0.20%
    C. 0.25%   D. 0.30%

32. Divestment is a combination of:
    A. Improved stone + gypsum bonded investment
    B. Improved stone + phosphate bonded investment
    C. Die stone+ ethyl silicate-bonded investment
    D. None of the above

33. Setting expansion of divestment is:
    A. 0.05%   B. 0.5%
    C. 0.9%   D. 0.01%

34. Plaster is manufactured by:
    A. Wet calcification
    B. Dry calcification
    C. Wet calcination
    D. Dry calcination

35. **Diagnostic cast is made up of:**
    A. Model stone
    B. Dental stone
    C. Improved stone
    D. Type V dental stone

36. **In comparison to plaster, particle size and shape of dental stone is/are:**
    A. Larger
    B. Irregular
    C. Both of the above
    D. None of the above

37. **One hour tensile strength of model plaster is:**
    A. 2.0 MPa
    B. 2.3 MPa
    C. 4.5 MPa
    D. 5.3 MPa

38. **By how much percentage setting expansion increases if setting gypsum products are immersed under water?**
    A. 0.01%
    B. 0.02%
    C. 0.1%
    D. 0.2%

Answers

1.B. Type I   Impression plaster

Type II   Plaster of Paris (Model plaster)

Type III   Medium strength stone

Type IV   High strength dental stone

Type V   High strength, high expansion dental stone.

2.C. $CaSO_4. 2H_2O$ 110-130°C $CaSO_{4. \frac{1}{2}} H_2O$ 130° –200°C $CaSO_4$

Gypsum $\longrightarrow$ Plaster or stone   Hexagonal anhydrite $\longrightarrow$

200-1000° C $\downarrow$

$CaSO_4.$
Orthorhombic anhydrite

3.C. Improved surface hardness of type IV dental stone makes it abrasion resistant during carving of wax pattern. (Rockwell hardness = 92)

4.C. This water powder ratio is less than that of type III and more than that of type V.

5.B. Type IV stone is required for making dies. The type IV stone is manufactured by calcining gypsum by boiling it in a 30% solution of calcium chloride ($CaCl_2$). It is also known as die stone.

6.C. This difference in solubility of dihydrate and hemihydrate is at room temperature (20°C) and is responsible for the setting reaction of gypsum products.

7.D. Greater the compactness of particles, lesser the water: powder ratio. Small amounts of surface-active materials reduce water: powder ratio. Finer the particles lesser the water: powder ratio.

8.B.   W:P ratio

Type I	0.50: 0.75
Type II	0.45 : 0.50
Type III	0.28 : 0.30
Type IV	0.22 : 0.24
Type V	0.18 : 0.22

9.A. Setting expansion at 2 hours

	Min (%)	Max (%)
Type I	0.00	0.15
Type II	0.00	0.30
Type III	0.00	0.20
Type IV	0.00	0.10
Type V	0.10	0.30

10.D. Compressive strength at 1hour (Psi)

Type I	580 ± 290
Type II	1300
Type III	3000
Type IV	5000
Type V	7000

11.A. Diameter of a Vicat needle is 1mm.

12.C. Weight of the small Gillmore needle is ¼ pound, and that of the large Gillmore needle is 1 pound.

13.D. Greater the mixing time and rate of spatulation, lesser will be the setting time. Setting time can be varied depending upon the quality and manufacturing process. If the temperature of mixture is above 50° C, longer is the setting time and at close to 100° C no reaction takes place.

14.B. Hexagonal anhydrite is the natural anhydrate. Its presence decreases the setting time.

15.B. At concentrations greater than 3.4% sodium sulfate acts as a retarder.

16.D. Inorganic salts act as accelerators though they may act as retarders above a certain concentration.

17.D. The citrates, acetates and borates generally retard the setting reaction; for a given anion, the particular cation employed appears to affect the retardation markedly. The accelerators and retarders regulate the setting time but also they generally reduce the setting expansion.

18.B. Retarders form a coating on the hemihydrate particles, thereby preventing them from going into solution in the usual manner 2% solution of borax. ($Na_2 B_4 O_7$. $10H_2o$) is a dependable retarded which delays setting by several hours.

19.A. It is 0.5 to 0.1% calcium sulfate dihydrate (terraalba), used by manufacturers to increase the speed of setting reaction.

20.A. This range depends upon the composition of the gypsum product regardless the type of the gypsum used.

21.C. With the addition of an accelerator, the time of interaction between dihydrate crystals is less, therefore, the outward thrust is less therefore expansion is less.

22.C. Regardless of the type of gypsum product employed an expansion of the mass can be detected the change from the hemihydrate to dihydrate. Depending upon the composition of the gypsum product this observed expansion may be as low as 0.06% linear to as high as 0.5%.

23.C. The wet strength is the strength when the water in excess of that required for the hydration of the hemihydrate is left in the test specimen. Wet strength is two or more time less than dry strength.

24.C. Both accelerators and retarders act as adulterants and reduce intercrystalline cohesion thereby reducing strength of dental stone.

25.B. Technically it may be considered as the time when the compressive strength is at least 80% of that attained at one hour most mordern product reach the ready for use state in 30 minutes.

26.C. Potato starch is present in soluble plaster. This potato starch make boundaries between plaster and cast. It make easy removal of cast from impression.

27.B. Rochelle salt is typical accelerator used to accelerate the setting of dental stone (type III gypsum product potassium sulfate is also a accelerator.

28.B. Dental stone (type III) has minimum 1 hour compressive strength of 3000 psi It is used for construction of cast in fabrication of full dentures that fit the soft tissue. The setting expansion of dental stone is 0.060 to 0.12%.

29.D. Dental stone, high strength (type IV) is also called die stone or densite or class II stone or improved stone. It has cuboidal shaped particle. The hardness is approximately 92 RHN.

30.D. Alphahemihydrate, potassium sulfate and borax are all constituents of dental stone.

31.D. Range of setting expansion of type V dental stone is 0.10-0.30%.

32.A. A commercial gypsum bonded material divestment is mixed with colloidal silica liquid since divestment is gypsum-bounded material it is not recommended for high fusing alloys.

33.C. The setting expansion of divestment is 0.9% and thermal expansion is 0.6% when it is heated to 667% C (1250% F). It is highly accurate technique for use with conventional gold alloy especially for extra-coronal preparation.

34.D. Strong heating is known as calcination. Plaster is manufactured by strong dry heating of calcium sulfate dihydrate.

35.A. As high strength is not required.

36.D. Dental stone is α type of hemihydrate and plaster is β hemihydrate. Stone has more small and regular particle size.

37.B. The tensile strength of plaster or stone is less affected by variations in the W/P ratio than is the compressive strength. However, the materials mixed at a high W:P ratios have tensile strengths as high as 25% of the corresponding compressive strength when the materials are mixed with low W:P ratios, the tensile strength is less than 10% of the corresponding compressive strength.

38.C. If stone cast is immersed in running water its linear dimension may decrease approximately 0.1% for every 20 minutes of such immersion. The gypsum of which the cast is composed is slightly soluble in water.

4 *Impression Materials*

1. Which of the following material/s is/are elastic in nature?
   A. Polyether
   B. Impression compound
   C. Both of the above
   D. None of the above

2. Which of the following impression materials is/are not thermostatic?
   A. Plaster of Paris
   B. Zinc oxide-eugenol
   C. Both of the above
   D. Impression compound

3. ADA specification number for impression compound is:
   A. 3
   B. 11
   C. 12
   D. 15

4. Which of the following applications is not used for type I impression compound?
   A. For making a primary impression
   B. For individual tooth impression
   C. To check undercut in inlay procedure
   D. None of the above

5. Major portion of impression compound is formed by:
   A. Carnuba wax
   B. Stearic acid
   C. Copal resin
   D. Coloring agent

6. Impression compound starts loosing its hardness at approximately:
   A. 29°C
   B. 39°C
   C. 49°C
   D. 59°C

7. Fusion temperature for impression compound is:
   A. 41.5°C
   B. 42.5°C
   C. 43.5°C
   D. 44.5°C

8. The linear contraction of impression compound from mouth temperature to room temperature of 25°C is:
   A. 0.1%
   B. 0.2%
   C. 0.3%
   D. 0.4%

9. Maximum flow of type I impression compound at $37°C$ is:
   A. 85%
   B. 70%
   C. 6%
   D. 2%

10. Which of the following is/are correct about type II impression compound?
    A. Flow not more than 85% at $37°C$
    B. Flow not less than 70% at $37°C$
    C. Both of the above
    D. None of the above

11. ADA specification number of zinc oxide-eugenol impression paste is:
    A. 23
    B. 15
    C. 18
    D. 16

12. Accelerator paste of zinc oxide-eugenol have all of the followings *except*:
    A. Polymerized resin
    B. Lanolin
    C. Fixed vegetable or mineral oil
    D. Resinous balsam

13. What is the function of polymerized resin in zinc oxide-eugenol paste?
    A. Retarder of the setting reaction
    B. Speeds the setting reaction
    C. Improves flow and mixing properties
    D. Acts as plasticizer

14. All of the followings are accelerators of zinc oxide-eugenol impression paste *except*?
    A. Calcium chloride
    B. Primary alcohol
    C. Glacial acetic acid
    D. None of the above

15. Initial setting time of type I impression paste is:
    A. 3 to 6 minutes
    B. 10 minutes
    C. 15 minutes
    D. 6 to 8 minutes

16. Which of the following factors increases the setting time of zinc oxide-eugenol impression paste?
    A. Acid coated zinc oxide particles
    B. Adding a drop of water
    C. Cooling the mixing slab
    D. Longer mixing time

17. According to ADA specification No. 16 the spread of type I impression paste is:
    A. 20 to 45 mm   B. 30 to 50 mm
    C. 10 to 35 mm   D. 40 to 55 mm

18. In non-eugenol paste, the zinc oxide reacts with:
    A. Carbolic acid   B. Diaminocaproic acid
    C. Carboxylic acid   D. Aminocaproic acid

19. Bite registration paste has all of the following properties *except*:
    A. Shorter setting time than ZOE impression paste
    B. More plasticizers than ZOE impression paste
    C. Both of the above
    D. None of the above

20. Particle size of hydrocolloids ranges from:
    A. 200 to 500 mm   B. 1 to 200 nm
    C. 300 to 500 nm   D. 500 to 800 nm

21. Gelation of agar and alginate is/are brought about by:
    A. Lowering the temperature
    B. Chemical reaction
    C. Both of the above
    D. None of the above

22. Gel strength of hydrocolloid is dependent on:
    A. Density of the fibrillar structure
    B. Filler particle
    C. Lowering the temperature
    D. All of the above

23. Sulfuric ester of a linear polymer of galactose is present in:
    A. Agar
    B. Alginate
    C. Elastomeric impression material
    D. Inelastic impression material

24. Percentage of thixotropic materials in agar is around:
    A. 13%–17%
    B. 1%–2%
    C. 0.5%–1.0%
    D. 0.2%–0.5%

25. Plasticizers of agar impression material include all *except*:
    A. Glycerine
    B. Thymol
    C. Both of the above
    D. None of the above

26. Temperature of storage section of agar impression material is:
    A. 100°C
    B. 65–68°C
    C. 46°C
    D. 55–58°C

27. Which of the followings acts as a gypsum hardener in alginate impression material?
    A. Zinc oxide
    B. Diatomaceous earth
    C. Potassium titanium fluoride
    D. Sodium phosphate

28. Maximum proportion by weight of alginate impression material, is formed by:
    A. Ester salts of alginic acid
    B. Calcium sulfate
    C. Zinc oxide
    D. Diatomaceous earth

29. Ideal gelation time for alginate impression material is:
    A. 1 to 2.0 minutes
    B. 2 to 2.5 minutes
    C. 3 to 4 minutes
    D. 4.5 to 5 minutes

30. Permanent deformation for alginate is:
    A. 0.12%
    B. 0.2%
    C. 1.2%
    D. 2.0%

31. Which of the following factors decrease(s) strength of alginate?
    A. Too much water
    B. Too little water
    C. Over mixing
    D. All of the above

32. Dustless alginate contains:
    A. Glycerol
    B. Glycol
    C. Glacial acetic acid
    D. Silica coated powder particles

33. Mixing time for fast set alginate is:
    A. 45 seconds
    B. 60 seconds
    C. 30 seconds
    D. 80 seconds

34. What should be the minimum thickness of the gel between the tray and the tissues in case of alginate?
    A. 1 mm   B. 3 mm
    C. 6 mm   D. 8 mm

35. For the disinfection of alginate impression, which of the following chemicals is/are used?
    A. Glutaraldehyde   B. Sodium hypochlorite
    C. Both of the above   D. None of the above

36. Rough or chalky stone cast is formed from alginate impression due to:
    A. Inadequate cleaning of impressions
    B. Excess water left in impressions
    C. Premature removal of cast
    D. All of the above

37. Grainy impression occurs by alginate due to:
    A. Inadequate mixing   B. Prolonged mixing
    C. Less water in mix   D. All of the above

38. What is the ADA specification number for elastomeric impression materials?
    A. 9   B. 25
    C. 19   D. 35

39. Which of the followings is present in reactor paste of polysulfide elastomeric impression material with maximum percentage by weight?
    A. Titanium oxide   B. Lead dioxide
    C. Dibutyl phthalate   D. Sulfur

40. Which of the followings is/are used as adhesive in case of elastomeric impression materials?
    A. Butyl rubber
    B. Acrylonitrile dissolved in a suitable volatile solvent, e.g. ether
    C. Both the above
    D. None of the above

41. By product of setting reaction of polysulfide impression material is:
    A. Ethyl alcohol   B. Water
    C. Oxygen   D. Any of the above

42. Which of the following elastomeric impression materials has highest permanent deformation?
    A. Polysulfide
    B. Condensation silicone
    C. Addition silicone
    D. Polyether

43. What should be the spacing between tray and tissue in case of polysulfide impression material?
    A. 1 mm
    B. 2 mm
    C. 4 mm
    D. 5 mm

44. Which of the following viscosities is not associated with condensation silicone?
    A. Light bodied
    B. Medium bodied
    C. Putty
    D. Heavy bodied

45. Catalyst in condensation silicone is:
    A. Colloidal silica
    B. Ortho ethyl silicate
    C. Stannous octate
    D. Dibutyl phthalate

46. Ethyl alcohol as a by-product is formed in:
    A. Polysulfide
    B. Condensation silicone
    C. Addition silicone
    D. Polyether

47. Polyvinyl siloxane is:
    A. Addition silicone
    B. Condensation silicone
    C. Polysulfide
    D. Polyether

48. Which of the followings is a by-product in addition silicone?
    A. Water
    B. Ethyl alcohol
    C. Hydrogen gas
    D. None of the above

49. Best dimensional stability among elastomers is of:
    A. Polyether
    B. Polysufide
    C. Condensation silicone
    D. Addition silicone

50. How much time gap can be given between impression making and pouring it in case of addition silicone?
    A. No time
    B. Half an hour
    C. One to two hours
    D. Up to 24 hours

51. Permanent deformation in case of addition silicone is:
    A. 0.01 to 0.03%   B. 0.03 to 0.05%
    C. 0.05 to 0.3%   D. 0.4 to 0.5%

52. Plasticizer in polyether rubber impression material is:
    A. Aromatic sulfonate ester
    B. Colloidal silica
    C. Glycolether
    D. Ortho ethyl silicate

53. Stiffest elastomeric impression material is:
    A. Polyether   B. Condensation silicone
    C. Polysulfide   D. Addition silicone

54. Which of the followings is hydrophilic in nature?
    A. Polysulfide   B. Addition silicone
    C. Polyether   D. Condensation silicone

55. Shelf-life of polyether impression material is:
    A. Less than one year
    B. More than two years
    C. Between one and two years
    D. None of the above

56. Reline technique is also known as:
    A. Single mix technique
    B. Multiple mix technique
    C. Two-stage putty-wash technique
    D. All of the above

57. Highest tear resistance is found in:
    A. Polysulfide
    B. Polyether urethane dimethacrylate
    C. Polyether
    D. Addition silicone

58. Which of the following improves flow and mixing properties
    of zinc oxide-eugenol paste?
    A. Zinc oxide
    B. Calcium chloride
    C. Canada and Peru balsam
    D. Fixed vegetable oil

Answers

1.A. Impression compound is an inelastic impression material.

2.D. Impression compound is a thermoplastic material, which softens on heating and hardens on cooling.

3.A. In the ADA specification No. 3 for type I dental impression compound, a maximum flow of 6% is allowable at mouth temperature. The flow should not be less than 85% at 45° C or (113° F).

4.D. Impression compound is used for all of the above 3 procedures.

5.C. Waxes or resins are the principal ingredients in the impression compound and comprise the matrix.

6.B. The glass transition temperature for impression compound is 39° C (102° F). Below glass transition temperature compound loses its fluid characteristics and has significant resistance to shear deformation.

7.C. The fusion temperature of impression compound is approximately 43.5° (110° F). The practical significance of the fusion temperature is that it indicates a definite reduction in plasticity during cooling. So, once the impression tray is seated it should be held firmly in position until the fusion temperature.

8.C. There is a resultant error due to this property, which is unavoidable

9.C. Refer to Answer No. 3.

10.D. ADA specification No. 3 type II compound is referred as tray compound. However the specification states further that the flow should not be less than 85% when temperature of impression compound is 45° C(113° F)

11.D. ADA specification No. 16 is for dental impression pastes or zinc oxide-eugenal impression paste two types of paste are designated type I hard and type II soft.

12.C. The fixed vegetable or mineral oil in ZOE paste act as plasticizer and it also aids in masking the action of eugenol as an irritant.

13.B. It also produces a smoother and more homogeneous product.

14.D. Calcium chloride, primary alcohols and glacial acetic acid all are accelerators of zinc oxide-eugend impression paste.

15.A. Initial setting time includes the mixing time, time for loading the tray and seating the tray in the mouth properly.

16.C. Cooling the mixing slab and spatula increases setting time but cooling should not be done below dewpoint.

17.B. According to ADA specification No. 16 the spread of type I impression paste is 30 to 50 mm. The proper proportion of two paste of same length one from each tube onto the mixing slab is taken. Mixing is continued for approximately 1 minute or until a uniform color of the mix is observed.

18.C. This is done to avoid the stinging or burning sensation produced by eugenol on soft tissues. The product produced is an insoluble "soap." The carboxylic acid generally used for dental purpose is orthoethoxy benzoic acid (EBA)

19.D. Plasticizers, such as petrolatum, are added to avoid adherence of material to tissues.

20.B. Somewhere between the extremes of the very small molecules in solution and the very large particle in suspension is the colloidal solution or colloidal sol. The size of particle are considered to be in the range of 1 to 200 nanometers (nm).

21.C. Gelation of agar is a reversible process and is temperature dependant. Gelation of alginate is a chemical reaction by formation of calcium alginate.

22.D. Greater the density of fibrillar structure, greater the strength of gel lower the temperature, greater the strength since increase in temperature causes increase in interfibrillar distance thus reducing cohesive forces. Filler particles render the brush heap structure more rigid and less flexible.

23.A. Agar, obtained form certain seaweeds, is chemically composed of a sulfuric ester of a linear polymer of galachose.

24.D. Percentage of thixotropic material in agar is 0.3 to 0.5%. The principle ingredient in agar by weight is water. The basic constituent of impression material is agar but it is by no means a main constituent by weight.

25.C. Thymol also acts as a bactericide.

26.B. It is evident that there is no satisfactory method for storing a hydrocolloid impression various storage media such as 2% potassium sulfate or 100% relative humidity have been suggested to prevent dimensional changes.

27.C. This produces on hard dense stone cast surface against the impression.

28.D. Diatomaceous earth acts as filler, and functions to:

- Increase strength and stiffness of the gel.
- Produce a smooth surface.
- Reduce tackiness.
- Form sol.

29.C. Probably the optimal gelation time is between 3 and 4 minutes at a room temprature of 20° C (68°F). The best method for measurement of gelation time is to observe the time from the start of mixing until the material is no longer adhesive when it is thumbed with clean, dry fingers.

30.C. For accurate result and to prevent dimensional changes the cast should be constructed immediately after the impression is obtained. There is no satisfactory method for storage of any of the hydrocolloid impression material.

31.D. Too much or too little water weakens the final gel making it less elastic. Over mixing breaks up the calcium alginate gel network as it is forming.

32.B. Some of the silica particles in the alginate impression material are of such a size and shape as to be a possible health hazard. So glycol 1% is use to make the powder dust free.

33.A. Gelation times is 1–2 minutes.

34.B. Taking the impression with alginate perforated tray and the tissue for either agar or alginate should always be at least 3 mm (1/8 inch).

35.C. Disinfections should be done for recommended immersion time (10 minutes) only to avoid distortion.

36.D. Rough or chalky stone cast is formed from alginate impression due to the following:

1. Inadequate cleaning of impression.

2. Excess water left in impression.

3. Premature removal of cast.

4. Leaving cast in impression for too long.

37.D. Grainy impression is due to the following:

1. Improper mixing.

2. Prolonged mixing.

3. Undue gelation.

4. Water/powder ratio too low.

38.C. Elastomeric impression materials are rubber like in nature. They are identified in ADA specification No. 19 as non-aqueous elastomeric dental impression materials.

39.B. Lead dioxide present in the reactor or catalyst paste acts as the oxidizing agent and produces the characteristic dark brown color.

40.C. It should be noted that the adhesive cements supplied with the rubber impression materials are not interchangeable.

41.B. One complete condensation reaction results in the release of three water molecules.

42.A. Polysufide has highest permanent deformation so for maximum accuracy stone die or cast should be constructed with in first 30 minutes after the removal of impression from the mouth.

43.B. For hydrocolloid impression greater bulk of material produces better accuracy. But for elastomers bulk should be less and it should be evenly distributed. The optimal thickness of impression is 2 to 4 mm.

44.B. ADA specification No. 19 provides four viscosities of silicone impression materials depending upon consistency. One of these is very heavy viscosity or putty. They are used as a tray material in conjunction with low viscosity silicone.

45.C. In condensation silicone cross-linking agent are tetraethyl orthosilicate and catalyst is stannous octoate. These reactions are at ambient temperatures, it is therefore, called room temperature vulcanization (RTV) silicone.

46.B. One complete condensation reaction of silicone results in the release of two molecules of ethyl alcohol.

47.A. In addition type silicone, base and catalyst pastes contain the vinyl silicone. In this case the polmerization is terminated with vinyl groups and cross-linked with hydride groups activated by the platinum salt catalyst.

48.C. This is not technically a by-product of the reaction but is produced only when proper proportions of vinyl silicone and hydride silicone are not maintained or impurities are present.

49.D. Addition silicones exhibit maximum dimensional stability because no reaction by-products are formed little residual polymerisation

50.D. This long time span can be afforded due to the high dimensional stability of the material.

51.C. Addition silicone impression materials are most dimensionally stable of all impression materials as no volatile by-product is released so there is no shrinkage. Therefore, the material remains dimensionally stable after removal from oral cavity.

52.C. In polyether rubbers, base contains polyether polymers, colloidal silica as filler and a plasticizer such as a glycolether or phthalate. Accelerator is alkyl aromatic sulfonate in addition to the filler and plasticizer.

53.A. Due to its high stiffness it is most difficult to remove this type of impression material from the undercuts.

54.C. The silicon impression materials have generals inherent hydrophobicity. But polyether is hydrophilic in nature. To render the surface of the impression hydrophilic surfactant is added to the paste. This surfactant then allows the impression material to wet soft tissue better and to be poured more easily.

55.B. This holds true only when the material is stored under normal environmental conditions.

56.C. Putty is used to form the intra-oral custom tray and wash material is placed in the putty impression and a final impression is made.

57.A. Excluding the very high viscosity putty class of rubbers the stiffness of the various kinds increases in following order: Polysulfide-condensation silicone-addition silicone-polyeter.

58.C. Canada balsam and Peru balsam are often used to increase flow and improve mixing properties. If the mixed paste is too thin or lacks body before it sets, filler such as kaolin talc may be added.

5   *Dental Waxes*

1. **Which of the followings is/are distillation products of petroleum?**
   - **A.** Paraffin wax
   - **B.** Microcrystalline waxes
   - **C.** Both of the above
   - **D.** None of the above

2. **Which of the following waxes occurs as a fine powder on the leaves of certain tropical palms:**
   - **A.** Candellila
   - **B.** Japan wax
   - **C.** Ouricury
   - **D.** Carnauba

3. **Which of the following waxes is used for casting pattern making?**
   - **A.** Boxing wax
   - **B.** Utility wax
   - **C.** Inaly wax
   - **D.** Corrective wax

4. **ADA specification number for dental wax is:**
   - **A.** 25
   - **B.** 4
   - **C.** 12
   - **D.** 18

5. **The minimum flow of inlay casting wax at 45°C should be:**
   - **A.** 60%
   - **B.** 70%
   - **C.** 6%
   - **D.** 100%

6. **Which of the following correctly describe type I inlay casting wax?**
   - **A.** Soft wax used for direct technique
   - **B.** Medium wax used for indirect technique
   - **C.** Soft wax used for indirect technique
   - **D.** Medium wax used for direct technique

7. **The maximum ingredient of inlay casting wax is:**
   - **A.** Paraffin wax
   - **B.** Carnauba wax
   - **C.** Ceresin
   - **D.** Gum dammar

8. **Which of the followings is added in inlay casting wax to improve the smoothness?**
   - **A.** Ceresin
   - **B.** Gum dammar
   - **C.** Candellila wax
   - **D.** Synthetic waxes

9. Maximum flow of type I inlay wax at 37°C is:
   A. 1%   B. 2%
   C. 3.5%   D. 3.0%

10. Minimum flow of type II inlay wax at 45°C is:
    A. 1%   B. 45%
    C. 70%   D. 85%

11. Coefficient of thermal expansion is highest for:
    A. Amalgam   B. Gold alloy
    C. Composite   D. Inlay casting wax

12. Major part of base plate wax is formed by:
    A. Paraffin   B. Beeswax
    C. Carnauba   D. Microcrystalline

13. Flow of corrective impression wax at 37°C should be:
    A. 70%   B. 1%
    C. 85%   D. 100%

14. Which of the followings is/are natural waxes?
    A. Carnauba wax   B. Ceresin
    C. Candellila wax   D. All of the above

15. All of the following are processing wax *except*:
    A. Base plate wax   B. Boxing wax
    C. Utility wax   D. None of the above

16. Which of the followings is added in inlay casting wax to decrease flow at mouth temperature?
    A. Paraffin wax   B. Carnauba wax
    C. Candellila wax   D. Ceresin

17. Which of the following factor/s is/are not responsible in releasing the stresses in inlay pattern?
    A. Contraction on cooling
    B. Occluded gas bubbles
    C. Change of shape of the wax during moulding
    D. None of the above

18. How much maximum percentage of total weight of wax pattern can be permitted to be present after vaporization?
    A. 0.1%   B. 0.01%
    C. 0.001%   D. 1.0%

19. **What is/are the function(s) of beeswax in inlay wax?**
    A. Decrease flow at mouth temperature
    B. Increase plasticity and increase moldability
    C. Provides smoothness
    D. Both A and C

20. **Base plate wax type I is used for:**
    A. Building veneers
    B. Making patterns to be tried in the oral cavity
    C. Trial filling in the oral cavity for warm climate in tropical countries
    D. None of the above

21. **Which of the following is an animal wax?**
    A. Crnauba wax
    B. Candellila
    C. Spermacetic wax
    D. Paraffin wax

22. **Which of the following is impression wax?**
    A. Inlay wax
    B. Casting wax
    C. Corrective wax
    D. Both A and B

23. **Which of the following is not an ideal requirement for an inlay casting wax?**
    A. There should be no flakiness or roughening of the surface when the wax is moulded after softening
    B. The flow should be more than 70% at 45°C
    C. The flow should be less than 1% at 37°C
    D. None of the above

24. **Flow of inlay wax is dependent on:**
    A. Temperature of wax
    B. Force applied
    C. The time the force is applied
    D. All of the above

25. **Percentage of carnauba wax in inlay casting wax is:**
    A. 40%
    B. 60%
    C. 25%
    D. 10%

26. **Which of the following method/s is/are used to avoid distortion of the wax?**
    A. Minimal carving and change in temperature
    B. Minimal storage of pattern
    C. Using warm instruments for carving
    D. All of the above

27. **Casting wax is supplied as:**
    A. Sheets only   B. Meshform only
    C. Both of the above   D. None of the above

28. **Which of the following types of base plate wax is used in mouth in normal climates?**
    A. Type II   B. Type I
    C. Type IV   D. Type III

29. **Percentage of bees wax in base-plate wax is:**
    A. 80%   B. 2.5%
    C. 3.0%   D. 12.0%

30. **Sticky wax consists of all of the followings *except*:**
    A. Yellow beeswax
    B. Rosin
    C. Gum dammar
    D. None of the above

31. **Corrective impression wax is used to:**
    A. Make functional impression of free end saddles
    B. Record posterior palatal seal in dentures
    C. Make functional impression for obturator
    D. All of the above

32. **Corrective impression wax consists of:**
    A. Paraffin
    B. Ceresin
    C. Both of the above
    D. Synthetic wax only

33. **How much percentage of eugenol is present in oil of clove?**
    A. 60%   B. 70%
    C. 95%   D. 45%

34. **Percentage of hard wax in agar is:**
    A. 3%   B. 0.5%–1.0%
    C. 2–3%   D. 0.1%

35. The purpose(s) of burn-out during casting procedure is/are:
    A. To eliminate the wax from the mould
    B. To expand the mould
    C. Both of the above
    D. None of the above

36. Which of the followings is/are a processing wax?
    A. Boxing wax   B. Bite registration wax
    C. Casting wax   D. All of the above

37. Which of the following properties of dental wax are higher than other dental materials?
    A. Elastic modulus
    B. Proportional limit
    C. Compressive strength
    D. None of the above

Answers

1.C. Paraffin wax is obtained from high boiling point fractions of petroleum. Microcrystalline waxes are obtained from heavier oil fractions of petroleum.

2.D. Carnauba wax occurs as a fine powder on the leaves of certain tropical palms. This wax is quite hard and has relatively high melting point. It also contributes to the glossiness of the wax surface.

3.C. The first procedure in the casting of an inlay or crown is the prepration of the wax pattern. If pattern is made in the tooth itself, it is a direct technique, if it is prepared on a die the procedure is called indirect technique.

4.B. ADA specification No. 4 for dental inlay casting wax type I is medium wax used in direct technique and type II is soft wax used in indirect technique.

5.B. The maximum flow permitted for type I waxes at 37° C is 1% in addition both type I and type II waxes must have a minimal flow of 70% at 45°C and maximum flow of 90%.

6.D. Refer to Answer No. 4.

7.A. Paraffin wax forms the major portion of inlay casting wax and provides the desired amount of mouldability (60%).

8.B. Gum dammar is also known as dammar resin. It also renders the wax resistant to cracking and flaking.

9.A. 37°C is the normal temperature of the oral cavity. A flow greater than 1% would cause distortion of the wax pattern during carving within the oral cavity.

10.C. A flow less than 70% would not render the wax plastic enough to flow into all areas of the preparation and produce a pattern with insufficient detail.

11.D. This is a disadvantage with waxes especially when they are being used in the direct technique of wax pattern fabrication.

12.A. Base-plate wax contains 75–80% paraffin wax.

13.D. Another group of dental waxes is composed of the impression wax also referred as bite or corrective wax they are quite soft at mouth temperature and do have sufficient body to register the details of soft tissue and they are rigid at room temperature. They are also known as impression or bite waxes.

14.D. Carnauba wax and candellila wax are of plant origin and ceresin is a hard mineral wax.

15.A. Processing waxes are used in various procedures as auxillary aids for example, boxing impressions before cast is poured.

16.B. Gum dammar increases the toughness of wax; carnauba wax is combined with paraffin to decrease the flow at mouth temperature. Candellila wax provides same general qualities as the carnauba wax. But its melting point is lower. So, it replaces carnauba wax.

17.D. Distortion is very probably the most serious problem to be faced when forming and removing the pattern from the mouth or die. It results from thermal changes and release of stresses. These stresses arise from contraction on cooling, change in shape during molding, carving, removal and time and temperature during storage.

18.A. The desirable properties of inlay casting wax is that on the temperature 400 to 500°C. It should vaporize from the mold without leaving solid residue. ADA specification allow resides not more than 0.1% of total weight of wax pattern.

19.B. Paraffin wax is 60%. It is main ingredient of inlay casting wax. Beeswax is 5% and it increases plasticity and moldability. Other ingredients are carnauba, ceresin, candellila wax.

20.A. Base-plate wax is of three types, type I is soft wax used for building veneers, type II is medium wax for making patterns and type III is hard wax for trial filling in the oral cavity for warm climate in tropical countries.

21.C. Carnauba wax, candellila wax ceresin, montanwax all are derived from mineral or vegetable sources. But spermacetic wax is derived from animal orgin.

22.C. Impression waxes are also called bite or corrective wax. They will distort if they are withdrawn from undercut area and therefore, have limited use in edentulous portion of mouth.

23.D. Refer to Answers No. 8, 9 and 10.

24.D. As temperature increases, flow also increases. If force applied is more, flow will increase. Flow is also directly proportional to the time of force application.

25.C. Percentage of carnauba wax in inlay casting wax is 25%. It's melting range is 84 to 91°C and it decreases flow at mouth temperature and contributes glossiness.

26.D. Most practical method for avoiding any possible delayed distortion is to invest the pattern immediately after removal from the mouth or the die. Once the investment hardens, there will be no more distortion of the pattern .

27.C. The casting wax is used for the same purpose as inlay wax in the formation of patterns mostly for metallic denture castings. These waxes are available in thin sheets and in readymade shape.

28.A. Refer to Answer No.20.

29.D. Base-plate wax is composed of mainly paraffin wax which is 75 to 85%, beeswax is 10 to 14% other waxes are carnauba wax synthetic wax, microcystalline wax.

30.D. Sticky waxes consist of yellow beeswax rosin, gum dammar. It is used to join or stabilize the pieces of broken material like dentures and costs. They also used to stabilize the components of a bridge before soldering.

31.D. Impression wax used generally in combination with other impression materials like ZOE, impression compound and polysulfide rubber. They are used to record non-undercut edentulous portions of the mouth.

32.C. Corrective impression wax consists of paraffin wax, ceresin wax, microcrystalline wax and synthetic wax.

33.B. Oil of clove contains 70-85% eugenol.

34.B. Hard wax in agar impression material acts as a filler.

35.C. The invested rings are placed in a room temperature furnace and heated to 900°F for gypsum-bonded investment during burnout wax is eliminated from mould and mould is expanded.

36.A. Refer to Answer No.15.

37.D. Elastic modulus proportional limit and compressive strength are lower to other dental materials but cofficient of thermal expansion is highest in waxes.

Introduction to Dental Resins

1. **Which of the following is not a use of synthetic resins?**
   A. Impression material B. Bonding
   C. Sealants   D. None of the above

2. **What should be the minimum molecular weight for a chemical to be considered a polymer?**
   A. 10,000   B. 5,000
   C. 2,000   D. 25,000

3. **Most of the dental resins are polymerized by:**
   A. Condensation polymerization
   B. Addition polymerization
   C. Both of the above
   D. None of the above

4. **The initiation energy for activation of each monomer molecular unit is:**
   A. 6000 to 8000 calories per mol
   B. 16,000 to 29, 000 calories per mol
   C. 25,000 to 32,000 calories per mol
   D. 500 to 5000 calories per mol

5. **Most denture base resins are polymerized by:**
   A. Heat activation   B. Chemical activation
   C. Light activation   D. None of the above

6. **Which of the following chemicals liberate free radicals during heat activation?**
   A. Benzoyl peroxide   B. Aromatic amine
   C. Camphoroquinone   D. Any of the above

7. **Which of the following is/are not used in light activated induction system?**
   A. Aromatic amines
   B. Camphoroquinone
   C. Both of the above
   D. None of the above

8. How much hydroquinone is used to retard polymerization during storage?
   A. 0.06%   B. 0.006%
   C. 0.6%   D. 0.01%

9. Which of the following is/are inhibitior (s) of polymerization?
   A. Impurities   B. Hydroquinone
   C. Oxygen   D. All of the above

10. Which of the following is not a type of copolymerization?
    A. Random type   B. Graft type
    C. Block type   D. None of the above

11. Which of the following is/are effects of cross-linking in polymerization in acrylic resins?
    A. Increased strength
    B. Increased water sorption
    C. Both of the above
    D. None of the above

12. Plasticizers are added to resins:
    A. To increase the solubility of the polymer in the monomer
    B. To decrease the brittleness of the polymer
    C. To decrease softening temperature
    D. All of the above

13. All of the following are a type of resin *except*:
    A. Polycarbonates
    B. Polyurethanes
    C. Both of the above
    D. None of the above

14. Boiling point of methyl methacrylate is:
    A. 15 °C   B. 21 °C
    C. 101.8 °C   D. 100.8 °C

15. Volume shrinkage of methyl methacrylate during polymerization is:
    A. 12.9%   B. 20.0%
    C. 21.0%   D. 9.12%

16. Density of methyl methacrylate is:
    A. 0.495 g/ml   B. 0.945 g/ml
    C. 0.549 g/ml   D. 0.465 g/ml

Answers

1.D. Synthetic resins are used as impression materials. For example, impression for post and core fabrication, as a sealant in cariogenic pits and fissures and as dentin bonding agents also.

2.B. Since any chemical compound having a molecular weight more than 5000 is classified as a macromolecule, therefore, synthetic resins are also macromolecules.

3.B. The resins employed extensively in dental procedures at the present time are produced by addition polymerization. The term polymerization when used alone is generally understood to indicate addition polymerization.

4.B. The induction or initiation period is the time during which the molecules of the initiator became activated and start to transfer their energy to the monomer molecules. The initiation energy for each monomers molecular unit is 16000 to 29000 calories per mole in the liquid phase.

5.A. Heat energy catalyzes the initiator benzoyl peroxide to split into free radicals, which react with the monomer.

6.A. As benzoyl peroxide liberates free radials, it acts as the initiator in synthetic resins.

7.D. Camphoroquinone–photoinitiator. Aromatic amine is dimethyle amino ethyl metharylate or accelerator or activator.

8.B. 0.006% or less of methyl ether of hydroquinone is used as inhibitor of polymerisation reaction.

9.B. Refer to Answer No. 8.

10.D. Random graft and block are all types of copolymerization.

11.C. These properties are altered due to formation of sufficient number of bridges between the linear macromolecules to form a three dimensional network.

12.D. Plasticizers are added to resin to reduce their fusion temperature. Plasticizers also increase the solubility of the polymer in the monomer and decrease the brittleness of the polymer. But plasticizers usually reduce the strength and hardness of the resin as well as the softening point.

13.D. Example of condensation polymerization are bakelite, polyurethane, polycarbonate, polysulfide rubber base impression material.

14.D. Methyl methacrylate is a clear, transparent liquid at room temperature. It's melting point is -48°C, boiling point is 100.8°C, density is 0.945 gram/ml at 20°C and heat of polymerization is 12.9 Kcal/ml.

15.C. A volume shrinkage of 21% occurs during the polymerization of the pure methylmethacrylate monomer and degree of polymerization varies with the condition of polymerization such as temperature, method of activation, type of initiator, purity of chemicals using polymer: monomer in 3:1 ratio, the volumetric shrinkage may be limited to approximately 6% (0.5% linear shrinkage).

16.B. This density is measured at 20° C. When methyl methacrylate monomer is polymerized to form poly (methyl methacrylate) the density of the mass changes from 0.94 to 1.19 g/cm^3.

1. **Bowen's resin is also known as:**
   A. Polyurethane
   B. Bis-GMA
   C. Polycarbonate
   D. Polymethyl methacrylate

2. **Which of the following is used as dentin bonding agent?**
   A. Hydroxy ethyl methacrylate
   B. Modified polyacrylic acid
   C. Penta acrylate monophosphate
   D. None of the above

3. **Density of polymethyl methacrylate is:**
   A. 0.19 g/cm^2
   B. 1.19 g/cm^2
   C. 2.19 g/cm^2
   D. 0.29 g/cm^2

4. **Knoop hardness number of polymethyl methacrylate is:**
   A. 16-18
   B. 18-20
   C. 20-22
   D. 23-25

5. **Cross-linking agent in polymethyl methacrylate is:**
   A. Hydroquinone
   B. Tertiary amine
   C. Glycol dimethacrylate
   D. Stable salts of sulfonic acid

6. **Liquid of heat activated polymethyl methacrylate contains all of the followings *except*:**
   A. Benzoyl peroxide
   B. Dibutyl phthalate
   C. Glycol dimethacrylate
   D. Hydroquinone

7. **Plasticizer in denture base acrylic resin is:**
   A. Dibutyl phthalate
   B. Glycol dimethacrylate
   C. Benzoyl peroxide
   D. Zinc or titanium oxide

8. **Polymer-monomer proportion of polymethyl methacrylate is:**
   A. 3:1 by volume
   B. 2:1 by weight
   C. Both of the above
   D. None of the above

9. Which of the following does not occur if low polymer-monomer ratio is used in case of polymethyl methacrylate?
   A. Greater polymerization shrinkage
   B. Dough stage will be difficult to manage
   C. More time is needed to reach the packing consistency
   D. Porosity can occur in denture

10. In which of the following stage acrylic resin can be packed into the mould?
    A. Rubbery stage   B. Stringy stage
    C. Gel stage   D. Stiff stage

11. Dough stage should remain mouldable for at least:
    A. 3 minutes   B. 5 minutes
    C. 10 minutes   D. 12 minutes

12. If material (denture base acrylic resin) is packed at rubbery or stiff stage, which of the following situations can occur?
    A. Increase in the vertical height of the denture
    B. Decrease in the vertical height of the denture
    C. Any one of the above
    D. Porosity in denture

13. Duration of 'Bench curing' is:
    A. 20 minutes   B. 30 minutes
    C. 90 minutes   D. 120 minutes

14. What is/are the advantage(s) of injection moulding technique?
    A. Dimensional accuracy
    B. Low free monomer content
    C. Good impact strength
    D. All of the above

15. Which of the following is present in chemically activated acrylic resin but absent in heat-activated acrylic resin?
    A. Glycol dimethacrylate
    B. Dibutyl phthalate
    C. Benzoyl peroxide
    D. Dimethyl-P-toluidine

16. Powder-liquid ratio of 'fluid resins' ranges from:
    A. 1:1 to 1.5:1   B. 2:1 to 2.5:1
    C. 3:1 to 3.5:1   D. 1:1 to 1.7:1

17. All of the following affect strength of polymethyl methacrylate *except*:
    A. Composition of resin
    B. Water sorption
    C. Degree of polymerization
    D. None of the above

18. Linear shrinkage of heat-cured acrylic resin is:
    A. 0.53%   B. 21%
    C. 0.26%   D. 80%

19. Linear shrinkage of self-cured acrylic resin is:
    A. 0.8%   B. 0.08%
    C. 0.26%   D. 0.53%

20. Coefficient of thermal expansion of acrylic resin is:
    A. $8 \times 10^{-6}/°C$ B. $10 \times 10^{-6}/°C$
    C. $81 \times 10^{-6}/°C$ D. $21 \times 10^{-6}/°C$

21. What is the percentage of residual monomer in heat cured acrylic resin?
    A. 0.1%   B. 0.4%
    C. 0.01%   D. 0.04%

22. What are the linear and volumetric contractions respectively if polymer and monomer are mixed in a ratio of 3:1 by volume?
    A. 6% and 0.5%   B. 21% and 6%
    C. 0.5% and 6%   D. 6% and 21%

23. Polymerization shrinkage is least in:
    A. Conventional acrylic resin
    B. High impact acrylic resin
    C. Vinyl acrylic resin
    D. Pour type of acrylic resin

24. Preformed crowns can be made up of:
    A. Polycarbonate   B. Cellulose acetate
    C. Aluminium   D. All of the above

25. Which of the following has the most natural appearance of all the preformed crowns?
    A. Cellulose acetate   B. Polycarbonate
    C. Aluminium   D. Tin-silver

26. Crazing can be avoided by:
    A. Using cross-linked acrylic
    B. Tinfoil separating media
    C. Metal moulds
    D. All of the above

27. Which of the following is not present in denture cleansers?
    A. Alkaline compound   B. Detergents
    C. Sodium perborate   D. None of the above

28. All of the following are true about resin denture teeth in comparison to porcelain denture teeth *except*:
    A. High fracture toughness
    B. Dimensionally stable because of absence of water resorption
    C. Cold flow under stress
    D. None of the above

29. Chemical bond to denture is present in:
    A. Porcelain teeth   B. Resin teeth
    C. Both of the above   D. None of the above

30. Which of the followings is/are a type of resilient liner(s)?
    A. Plasticized acrylic resin
    B. Vinyl resin
    C. Silicone rubbers
    D. All of the above

31. Room temperature-vulcanized (RTV) silicones resemble:
    A. Condensation silicone
    B. Addition silicone
    C. Both of the above
    D. None of the above

32. Most recent material in maxillofacial prosthesis is:
    A. Polymethyl methacrylate
    B. Plasticized polyvinylchloride
    C. Room temperature vulcanizing silicone
    D. Polyurethane polymers

33. Custom made crowns are made up of:
    A. Polyethyl methacrylate resins
    B. Epimine resins
    C. Microfilled composite resins
    D. All of the above

Answers

1.B. The backbone of the molecule formed in the system of acrylic resin is similar to the epoxy resin but functional reactive groups are acrylic. This resin is known by Bis-GMA and is an aromatic ester of dimethacrylate.

2.C. In dentin bonding agent phosphate group bond to calcium during dentin priming and during polymerization. Methacrylate group reacts with composite material making bond between composite and dentin.

3.B. Poly (methyl methacrylate) is a transparent resin of remarkable clarity, its specific gravity is 1.19, and tensile strength is approximately 59 MPa.

4.B. Poly (methyl methacrylate) is chemically stable to heat. It will soften at 125 degree C and it can be molded as a thermoplastic material. It is hard resin with a knoop hardness number of 18 to 20.

5.C. Many acrylic resin denture base materials contain a cross-linking agent such as glycol dimethacrylate. The polymer is cross-linked through CH_2-CH_2 group in at least two directions to form a bridged network. Cross-linking agents are incorporated into the liquid component at a concentration at 1 to 2 vol%.

6.A. Benzoyl peroxide is the initiator and is added to the powder (polymer).

7.A. This is the internal plasticizer since the plasticizing agent is a part of the polymer.

8.C. The proper polymer to monomer ratio is generally 3:1 by volume and 2:1 by weight. Failure to blend properly the powder and liquid can result in low strength, porosities and poor color in denture.

9.B. In general the more polymer is used, the shorter will be the reaction time. Furthermore the shrinkage of the resin will be lower.

10.C. Gel stage is also known as the dough stage.

11.B. Five minutes is the working time for denture base resins during which they remain in dough stage and can be packed into the mould cavity.

12.A. Rubbery and stiff stages are reached after dough stage and the material no longer remains mouldable hence, cannot be packed properly into the mould.

13.B. For bench curing, flask is removed from water and cooled on the bench for 30 minutes and then immersed in cold water for 15 minutes and then denture is removed from the flask.

14.D. Advantage of the injection molding technique over the usual compression molding method is that no trial closure is necessary as the mold is properly filled automatically. However, no difference between the two methods in accuracy or physical properties is obtained.

15.D. Dimethyl-P-toluidine is the tertiary amine, which acts as the initiator in chemically cured resins.

16.B. This ratio is less than the polymer-monomer ratio of resins used in compression molding technique, i.e. 3:1.

17.D. The strength of resin is reduced after the sorption of water. Decrease degree of polymerization result in decrease in strength and rigidity. Strength is also reduced by finishing and polishing with abrasive agents.

18.A. The processing shrinkage has been measured as 0.53% for heat cured resin as compared with only 26% for self-cured resin.

19.C. Refer Answer No. 18.

20.C. Coefficient of thermal expansion of acrylic resin is 81×10^{-6} per degree C. The impact strength of the heat-cured resin is 0.98 to 1.27 Joules, and for self-cured resin is 0.78 Joules.

21.B. Percentage of free monomer in heat-cured acrylic resins is 0.2 to 0.5%. Chemically cured acrylic resins generally display 3 to 5% free monomer.

22.C. On the basis of probable volumetric shrinkage resin denture base should shrink linearly more than 2%. Thermal shrinkage of the resin is the chief contributor to the linear shrinkage phenomenon.

23.B. Polymerization shrinkage:

- Conventional acrylic resin 0.43%

- High impact acrylic resin 0.12%

- Vinyl acrylic resin 0.33%

- Pour type of acrylic resin 0.48%

24.D. Temporary crown and bridge material may be preformed or custom made. Example of preformed crowns are polycarbonate crown, cellulose acetate, aluminum and tin-silver crowns.

25.B. Polycarbonate crown has natural appearance and is commonly use in children.

26.D. Relaxation of surface stresses may result in the formation of cracks or crazing. Crazing may indicate the beginning of a fracture. Crazing can be avoided by using cross-linked agent, separating media, and metal mould.

27.D. Composition of denture cleansers:

- Alkaline compound

- Detergent

- Sodium perborate

- Flavouring agent.

28.B. Water absorption exerts significant effects on the properties of denture base resins. In case of polymethyl methacrylate its value is 0.69 mg/cm^2.

29.B. Resin teeth and denture base resin both have same basic chemical composition therefore, chemical bonding occurs between resin teeth and resin denture base.

30.D. The type of acrylic soft or resilient liners are: (1) plasticized acrylic resin, (2) vinyl resin (3) silicon rubbers (4) polyurea-thane and poly phosphazine rubber.

31.A. Room temperature vulcanizing silicone or RTV silicone is condensation type silicone. It is transparent and its prosthesis can be easily fabricated in dental laboratory. But RTV is not as strong as heat-vulcanized silicone.

32.D. Polyurethane polymers polymerize at room temperature, give a life like appearance but are subject to deterioration.

33.D. Custom made crowns are made up of:

1. Polymethyl methacrylate resin.

2. Microfilled composite resin.

3. Epimine resins.

4. Polyethyl (isobutyl methacrylate resins).

8 Introduction to Tooth Colored Restorative Materials

1. **Disadvantages of glass ionomer is/are:**
   A. Inferior esthetic quality as compared to composite
   B. Low strength
   C. Very sensitive to manipulation
   D. All of the above

2. **Amine accelerator in light activated resin is:**
   A. Camphoroquinone
   B. Hydroquinone
   C. Diethyl-amino-ethyl-methacrylate
   D. All of the above

3. **Which of the followings are advantages of hybrid composite materials?**
   A. Improved physical property
   B. Better finishing than conventional composite
   C. Abrasion resistance between conventional and microfilled composite
   D. All of the above

4. **How many times strength of porcelain is increased if it is reinforced with alumina crystals?**
   A. Two times   B. Three times
   C. Four times   D. Eight times

5. **Platinum tin foil adaptation is effective:**
   A. In improving the esthetics
   B. In maintaining the esthetics
   C. Both of the above
   D. None of the above

6. **Which of the following layers is formed in platinum tin foil adaptation?**
   A. Chromium layer   B. Oxide layer
   C. Hydroxide layer   D. Nitrate layer

7. The minimum occlusal reduction for castable ceramic should be:
   A. 1.5 mm
   B. 2.0 mm
   C. 1.0 mm
   D. 3 mm

8. The minimum proximal reduction in case of castable ceramic should be:
   A. 2.0 mm
   B. 1.5 mm
   C. 1.0 mm
   D. 2.25 mm

9. Contraindications to Maryland bridge include all *except*:
   A. Large restorations
   B. Insufficient bonding area
   C. Poor alignment of abutments
   D. None of the above

10. Preconditioning treatment of metal cast is done by:
    A. Sulfuric acid
    B. Hydrogen chloride
    C. Ammonium hydroxide
    D. Phosphoric acid

11. Which of the following solutions is/are used for electrolytic etching of metal cast restorations?
    A. Nitric acid
    B. Glacial acetic acid
    C. Both of the above
    D. None of the above

12. Cleaning agent used for metal cast restorations is:
    A. Nitric acid
    B. Phosphoric acid
    C. Hydrogen chloride
    D. Sulfuric acid

13. Which of the following is not a feature of silicate cement?
    A. Acidity of cement for one week
    B. Microleakage increases with age
    C. Both of the above
    D. None of the above

14. What is the least thickness of remaining pulpal dentin for the use of silicate cement?
    A. 2.0 mm
    B. 2.5 mm
    C. 3.0 mm
    D. 3.5 mm

15. In post-retained restorations what should be length of the post?
    A. Double of the crown length
    B. Half of the crown length
    C. One-third of the crown length
    D. Almost equal to the crown length

16. What should be the diameter of the post in post-retained restoration?
    A. One-third of diameter of the root treated
    B. Half of diameter of the root treated
    C. One-fourth of diameter of the root treated
    D. Between A and C

17. Glass ionomer cement forms permanent adhesive bond to:
    A. Enamel only
    B. Dentin only
    C. Both of the above
    D. None of the above

18. Laminated restoration utilizes:
    A. Zinc phosphate cement
    B. Glass ionomer cement
    C. Both of the above
    D. None of the above

Answers

1.D. Composites can be color matched. It has low strength. Sensitive to moisture contamination.

2.C. Light activated resin has diethyl-amino-ethyl-methacrylate as accelerator and camphoroquinone as photoinitiator.

3.D. Because of their surface smoothness and reasonably good strength, hybrid composites are widely used for anterior restorations, including class IV sites and stress-bearing restorations.

4.A. Aluminous porcelain is used to strengthen the overlying enamel porcelain and to resist deepening of microcracks.

5.C. Bonding aluminous porcelain to platinum foil copings makes use of tin oxide coatings on platinum foil. The bonded foil would act as an inner skin on the fit surface to reduce subsurface porosity and formation of microcracks in the porcelain, thereby increasing the fracture resisitance of the unit.

6.B. The oxide layer is formed on the outer foil, which becomes a part of the crown. This helps in improving esthetics.

7.B. Two mm is the minimum thickness required to provide sufficient strength to castable ceramic to bear the average occlusal load.

8.B. On proximal surface thickness of 1.0 mm is sufficient to provide required strength.

9.D. In case of insufficient bonding area and poor alignment of abutment teeth improper bonding is achieved.

10.C. Five percent ammonium hydroxide is used for 5 minutes and then rinsed.

11.C. A solution of 98 ml 0.1N nitric acid and 2 ml of glacial acetic acid is used. A current of 400 MA/cm^2 is used.

12.C. 18% hydrochloric acid is used for 10 minutes, by vibrating in an ultrasonic vibrator.

13.D. Acidity of silicate cement remains high for one week (pH is less than 3 at the time of insertion and remains below seven even after 1 month). Silicate cements degrade over time and so does the microleakage.

14.C. For other cements, remaining dentin thickness can be 2 mm but due to silicate cement's severe irritant action on the pulp, remaining dentin thickness should be at least 3 mm.

15.D. The length of the post in post-retained restorations should be almost equal to crown length for proper retention and stability.

16.D. The diameter of the post also depends upon the following:

1. Occlusal load on the tooth.
2. Strength of the material used to fabricate the post.
3. Condition of the remaining portion of the tooth currently for the materials used for the fabrication of the post the thickness of between one-fourth to one-third diameter provide sufficient strength.

17.C. Glass ionomer cement bonds to both enamel and dentin by the chelation of the carbonyl groups of acids with the calcium in the apatite of enamel and dentin.

18.B. Laminated restorations utilize glass ionomer as lining material for composite resins.

9   Dental Materials for Pulp Protection

1. **Which of the following is not a component of liquid of dental cements?**
   A. Modified phosphoric acid
   B. Chelating agent
   C. Polyacrylic acid
   D. None of the above

2. **Which of the followings cements is/are used as an intermediate restorative material?**
   A. Zinc phosphate   B. Polycarbonates
   C. Both of the above   D. None of the above

3. **Thickness of varnishes should be:**
   A. 0.01 mm   B. 0.1 mm
   C. 1.0 mm   D. 0.25 mm

4. **Copal resin varnish contains:**
   A. 10% Copal resins and 90% ether
   B. 20% Copal resins and 80% ether
   C. 15% Copal resins and 85% ether
   D. 25% Copal resins and 75% ether

5. **Varnishes should not be used under restoration of:**
   A. Glass ionomer cement
   B. Composite
   C. Resin modified glass ionomer
   D. All of the above

6. **Cavity liners act as barrier agent for:**
   A. Passage of irritants   B. Thermal sensitivity
   C. Both of the above   D. None of the above

7. **Which of the following is not an objective of high strength base?**
   A. To protect pulp from various irritants
   B. To encourage recovery of the injured pulp
   C. To provide mechanical support for the pulp
   D. None of the above

8. What is the maximum thickness of light cure glass ionomer cement to cure at a time?
   A. 1.0 mm
   B. 0.5 mm
   C. 1.2 mm
   D. 2.0 mm

9. Ionic bonding is found in:
   A. Glass ionomer cement
   B. Polycarboxylate cement
   C. Zinc phosphate cement
   D. All of the above

10. Crystalline matrix is found in:
    A. Polycarboxylate cement
    B. Glass ionomer cement
    C. Both of the above
    D. Zinc phosphate cement

11. Calcium hydroxide liner consists of all of the following *except*:
    A. Zinc stearate
    B. Glycol salicylate
    C. Calcium tungstate
    D. None of the above

12. Calcium hydroxide arrests carious process by:
    A. Neutralizing the acid
    B. Hardening softened dentin
    C. Remineralizing softened dentin
    D. All of the above

13. Treatment of exposed vital pulp is:
    A. Indirect pulp capping
    B. Direct pulp capping
    C. Pulpotomy
    D. Both B and C

14. Treatment of choice for deep seated caries is:
    A. Direct pulp capping
    B. Pulpotomy
    C. Pulpectomy
    D. Indirect pulp capping

15. pH of non-eugenol temporary cement is:
    A. 6
    B. 7
    C. 8
    D. 9

16. Action of zinc oxide-eugenol on dentin is:
    A. Irritating
    B. Sedative
    C. Can be both
    D. None of the above

17. **Type I zinc oxide-eugenol cement is used for:**
    A. Sedation of pulp
    B. Temporary dressings
    C. Restorations
    D. Temporary cementation

18. **Least percentage of which of the followings is found in zinc oxide-eugenol cement?**
    A. Zinc oxide
    B. White resin
    C. Zinc stearate
    D. Olive oil

19. **Type III ZOE is used in:**
    A. Temporary cementation
    B. Permanent cementation
    C. Temporary filling
    D. Cavity liner

20. **Type of ZOE used for cavity liner is:**
    A. Type II
    B. Type III
    C. Type IV
    D. Type I

Answers

1.D. Modified phosphoric acid is a constituent of liquid of zinc phosphate cement. Chelating agent and polyacrylic acid are constituents of glass ionomer cement.

2.C. Intermediate restorations are the secondary use of zinc phosphate and zinc polycarboxylate cements.

3.B. This thickness of varnish should be attained in layer applications since as one layer dries small pin holes develop, therefore, two to three applications are recommended.

4.A. Copal resin is the natural gum. Solvents that can be used are ether, chloroform, acetone, alcohol or benzene.

5.D. In case of resin restorations, they cause softening of the resin and prevent proper wetting by the bonding agent. They also prevent adhesion of GIC to dentin.

6.C. They prevent passage of microorganisms and their by-products and oral fluids into the dentinal tubules.

7.D. High strength bases, besides providing mechanical support, protect pulp from various irritants and might encourage recovery of pulp by promoting secondary dentin formation.

8.D. With the light-cured GIC, conditioning of the dentine surface, such as with polyacrylic acid, is not required. However, thicknesses greater than 2 mm do not cure adequately.

9.C. Polycarboxylate and glass ionomer cement both show covalent bonding.

10.D. Polycarboxylate and glass ionomer cement, both form an amorphous matrix.

11.D. The main purpose of cavity liners is to use the beneficial effects of calcium hydroxide in accelerating the formation of reparative dentine. This type of liner not be left on the margins of the cavity preparation.

12.D. The alkaline nature of calcium hydroxide neutralizes the acid. Remineralization of carious softened dentin can be accomplished by means of calcium hydroxide.

13.D. Direct pulp capping is indicated for pin-point pulp exposures. Pulpotomy is mostly done in case of deciduous teeth or permanent teeth with incompletely formed roots.

14.D. Indirect pulp capping is done when pulp has not been exposed.

15.B. Substitution of a portion of the eugenol with orthoethoxy benxoic acid results in an appreciable increase in strength as does the incorporation of polymers.

16.B. The sedative action is due to the eugenol content.

17.D. Type I zinc oxide-eugenol cement is used for temporary cementation of restorations.
Type II permanent cementation of restorations or appliances.
Type III temporary dressings and thermal insulating bases.
Type IV cavity liners.

18.C. Zinc stearate is used as a plasticizer. While resin reduces brittleness.

19.C. Refer to Answer No. 17

20.C. Refer to Answer No. 17

10   *Luting Cements*

1. Desired compressive strength for temporary cementation is:
   - **A.** 25 MPa
   - **B.** 30 MPa
   - **C.** 35 MPa
   - **D.** 40 MPa

2. What is the percentage of staybelite resin in Grossman cement?
   - **A.** 68%
   - **B.** 48%
   - **C.** 27%
   - **D.** 15%

3. Film thickness of type I zinc phosphate cement should not be more than:
   - **A.** 25 µm
   - **B.** 40 µm
   - **C.** 35 µm
   - **D.** 50 µm

4. Which of the following add in sintering of zinc phosphate cement?
   - **A.** Zinc oxide
   - **B.** Magnesium oxide
   - **C.** Bismuth trioxide
   - **D.** Barium oxide

5. Which of the following act as buffer to reduce rate of reaction?
   - **A.** Magnesium oxide
   - **B.** Aluminum phosphate
   - **C.** Phosphoric acid
   - **D.** Calcium oxide

6. According to ADA specification, what should be maximum level of solubility for zinc phosphate cement?
   - **A.** 0.6 wt%
   - **B.** 0.06 wt%
   - **C.** 6.0 wt%
   - **D.** 0.1 wt%

7. Hopeite is:
   - **A.** $Al_2(PO_4)_3 . 4H_2O$
   - **B.** $Na_3 PO_4 . 4H_2O$
   - **C.** $Zn_3 (PO_4)_2 . 4H_2O$
   - **D.** $Zn_3(PO_4)_2 . 3H_2O$

8. All of the following factors increase setting time of zinc phosphate cement *except*:
   - **A.** Presence of excess water
   - **B.** Higher the temperature
   - **C.** Both of the above
   - **D.** None of the above

9. Type III zinc silicophosphate cement is used for:
   A. Cementing media
   B. Temporary posterior filling material
   C. Both of the above
   D. None of the above

10. Major portion of glass ionomer cement powder is formed by:
    A. Al_2O_3
    B. SiO_2
    C. AlF_3
    D. CaF_2

11. Bond strength of glass ionomer to tooth structure is:
    A. 1-5 MPa
    B. 6-16 MPa
    C. 16-26 MPa
    D. 25-30 MPa

12. Which of the following bonds is/are formed by glass ionomer to tooth structure?
    A. Chemical
    B. Micromechanical
    C. Both of the above
    D. None of the above

13. Glass ionomer cement is:
    A. Bacteriostatic
    B. Bacteriocidal
    C. Both of the above
    D. None of the above

14. Type I glass ionomer cement is used for:
    A. Cementation
    B. Lining
    C. Base
    D. All of the above

15. Miracle mix is:
    A. Type I glass ionomer + admixed silver amalgam alloy
    B. Type II glass ionomer + spherical silver amalgam alloy
    C. Type II glass ionomer + admixed silver amalgam alloy
    D. Type I glass ionomer + spherical silver amalgam alloy

16. Which of the following types of initiator is/are present in powder of dual cure glass ionomer cement?
    A. Light cure initiator only
    B. Chemical cure initiator only
    C. Both of the above
    D. Any one of A and B

Answers

1.C. Because the restorations will ultimately be removed, the maximum allowable strength, according to ADA specification No. 30, is 35 MPa.

2.C. Composition of Grossman's sealer:
Powder: Zinc oxide reagent 42%
Staybelite resin 27%
Bismuth subcarbonate 15%
Barium sulfate 15%
Sodium borate (anhydrous) 1%
Liquid: Eugenol or oil of pimeta leaf.

3.A. A thinner film has fever internal flaws compared with a thicker one. ADA specification No. 8 recommends maximum film thickness of 25 µm for type I cements (Dental cements for bonding applications).

4.B. Zinc oxide (90%) and magnesium oxide (10%) are sintered at temperatures between 1000°C and 1400°C into a cake that is subsequently ground into a fine powder.

5.B. This reacts with the zinc present in solution to form zinc aluminophosphate gel.

6.B. The solubility rate of zinc phosphate cement is appreciably greater in dilute organic acids (e.g. lactic, acetic and particularly citric). With the exception of resin cements, all the cements have the potential for significant degradation in oral fluids.

7.C. Zinc phosphate tetrahydrate.

8.C. Greater the amount of water, more will be the rate of ionization of the acid therefore, faster will be acid base reaction. Decrease in temperature increases setting time.

9.C. Indications for use of zinc silicophosphate cement are similar to those of zinc phosphate cement.

10.B. The glass ionomer powder is an acid-soluble calcium fluoroaluminosilicate glass. The particles of the powder are in the range of 20 to 50 μm. It also contains 26% of fluoride compounds.

11.B. The bond to enamel is always higher than that to dentine, probably because of the greater inorganic content of enamel and its greater homogeneity.

12.C. The micromechanical type of bonding of GIC to tooth structure takes place in case of resin modified glass ionomer cement. Chemical bonding occurs by chelation of carbonyl groups of polyacids with calcium of enamel and dentin.

13.C. Fluoride is released from GIC into an aqueous medium for an indefinite period. Fluoride inhibits carbohydrate metabolism by acidogenic plaque microflora. Fluoride enters microorganism and induces enzyme inhibition, leading to a slower rate of acid production.

14.D. Type I glass ionomer cement is used for luting purposes.

15.B. It is also called as silver alloy admix.

16.C. Dual cure resin cement systems use both chemical and light activation.

11

Bonding and Acid Etch Technique

1. **Glass ionomer with composite is known as:**
   A. Miracle mix
   B. Cermet
   C. Compomer
   D. None of the above

2. **Which of the following is/are secondary chemical bond?**
   A. Ionic bond
   B. Covalent bond
   C. Both of the above
   D. Hydrogen bond

3. **Which of the following bonds is formed by a shared common pool of valence electrons contributed by all atoms?**
   A. Covalent bond
   B. Hydrogen bond
   C. van der Waals forces
   D. Metallic bond

4. **The length of macrotags is:**
   A. 0.1 to 1.0 μm
   B. 1.0 to 2.0 μm
   C. 2.0 to 5.0μm
   D. 5.0 to 8.0 μm

5. **Dental bonding is primarily bonded on:**
   A. Mechanical bonding
   B. Chemical bonding
   C. Both of the above
   D. None of the above

6. **Maximum size of micro-mechanical bonding is:**
   A. 1 μm
   B. 10 μm
   C. 100 μm
   D. 5 μm

7. **Which of the followings has lowest shear strength?**
   A. Enamel
   B. Dentin
   C. Composite
   D. Amalgam

8. **Most commonly used etching agent is:**
   A. 47% phosphoric acid
   B. 35% hydrochloric acid
   C. 37% sulfuric acid
   D. 37% phosphoric acid

9. **Normal etching time is:**
   A. 10 minutes
   B. 15 minutes
   C. 20 minutes
   D. None of the above

10. **Type of bonding between etched enamel and enamel bonding agent is:**
    A. Mechanical bonding
    B. Chemical bonding
    C. Both of the above
    D. None of the above

11. **Which of the following is/are absent in enamel bonding agent?**
    A. Bis-GMA
    B. TEG-DMA
    C. Both of the above
    D. None of the above

12. **Which of the following is/are absent in dentin bonding agent?**
    A. Bis-GMA
    B. Triethyl glycol dimethacrylate
    C. Both of the above
    D. None of the above

13. **Dentin bonding agent should contain:**
    A. Hydrophilic part
    B. Hydrophobic part
    C. Both of the above
    D. None of the above

14. **Acid etching was developed by:**
    A. Smith
    B. GV Black
    C. Buonocore
    D. Aristotle

15. **Most important property of sealant is:**
    A. To be hydrophobic in nature
    B. To be hydrophilic in nature
    C. To flow into narrow pits and fissures
    D. None of the above

16. **Which of the following is/are beneficial property/ies of sealant to adapt more closely to enamel surface?**
    A. High coefficient of penetration
    B. High surface tension
    C. Low viscosity
    D. All of the above

17. **Use of phosphoric acid more than etching concentration leads to formation of:**
    A. Dicalcium phosphate
    B. Monocalcium phosphate monohydrate
    C. Tricalcium phosphate
    D. None of the above

18. **At which concentration of phosphoric acid monocalcium phosphate is formed?**
    A. 37%
    B. 47%
    C. 50%
    D. 27%

19. **Mode of action of acid etching is/are:**
    A. Creation of microporosities
    B. Increase in surface area
    C. Increase in surface energy
    D. All of the above

20. **Tooth with high fluoride content requires:**
    A. Less etching time   B. More etching time
    C. Can not be etched   D. Same etching time

21. **Highest bond strength of etched enamel with latest adhesive composites is:**
    A. 16 MPa   B. 8 MPa
    C. 25 MPa   D. 52 MPa

Answers

1.C. A light cured glass ionomer can be described as a combination of both addition polymerization and acid base reactivity, yielding a so-called hybrid material compomer, because it combines some of the composite material properties with those of the glass ionomers.

2.D. In contrast with primary bonds, secondary bonds do not share electrons. Instead charge variations among molecules or atomic groups include polar forces that attract the molecules. van der Waals forces also is a secondary bond.

3.D. Because of their ability to donate and recover electrons, atoms in a metal crystal exist as clusters of positive metal ions surrounded by the gas of electrons. This structure is responsible for the excellent electrical and thermal conductivity of metals and also for their ability to deform plastically.

4.C. Resin tags that formed between enamel rod peripheries are called macrotags. Smaller tags are formed across the end of each rod where individual hydroxy-apatite crystals have been dissolved, leaving crypts outlined by residual organic material. These fine tags are called microtags. Macrotags and microtags are the basis for enamel micro-mechanical bonding.

5.A. Except for cements like glass ionomer cement (which chelates with calcium of hydroxyapatite), dental bonding is mainly of mechanical type.

6.B. Almost every case of dental adhesion is based primarily on mechanical bonding. If the mechanical roughness produces a microscopically interlocked adhesive and adhererend with dimensions of less than approximately 10 µm, then the situation is described as micro-mechanical bonding (micro-mechanical retention or microretention).

7.C. Shear strength values:

Enamel	85-205
Dentin	160-180
Composites	25-125
Silver amalgam	115-135

8.D. Concentration range for phosphoric acid used in acid etching is 30 to 50%. Concentration greater than 50% lead to the formation of monocalcium phosphate monohydrate on the etched surface that inhibits further dissolution.

9.D. Length of time for application of etchant is often 15 seconds.

10.A. This occurs by formation of resin tags which penetrate into the enamel surface.

11.D. Both Bis-GMA and TEG-DMA are present in enamel bonding agents to control viscosity.

12.C. Dentin bonding agents contain NPG-GMA (a condensation product of N-Phenyl glycine and glycidyl methacrylate) or HEMA (Hydroxy ethyl methacrylate).

13.C. The hydrophilic part will displace the dentinal fluid in the tubules and form a resin tag and the hydrophobic part will bond with the composite resin.

14.C. Application of 50% phosphoric acid for 60 seconds results in formation of a monocalcium phosphate monohydrate precipitate that can be rinsed off. However, concentrations below 27% may create a dicalcium phosphate monohydrate precipitate that cannot be easily removed and, consequently may interfere with adhesion.

15.C. The objective of sealant use is for the resin to penetrate into the pits and fissures and to polymerize and seal these areas against the oral bacteria and debris.

16.D. To enhance wetting and mechanical retention of the sealant, the tooth surface is first conditioned by etching with acids.

17.B. Refer to Answer No. 14

18.C. Refer to Answer No.14

19.D. The formation of resin microtags within the enamel surface is the fundamental mechanism of adhesion of resin to enamel. The bond strengths of composite of phosphoric acid-etched enamel usually exceed 20 MPa.

20.B. Primary tooth also requires a longer etching time.

21.C. A Bis-GMA-triethylene glycol dimethocrylate (TEG-DMA) resin tends to yield lower values, whereas some of the newer enamel and dentine bonding agents can yield large values.

1. Creep percentage of low copper alloy is:
   - A. 2.0%
   - B. 0.4%
   - C. 0.13%
   - D. 0.23%

2. Lowest percentage of zinc necessary to cause delayed expansion in amalgam is:
   - A. 0.1%
   - B. 0.02%
   - C. 0.2%
   - D. 0.01%

3. How much minimum time is needed by dental amalgam to bear the average masticatory forces?
   - A. One hour
   - B. Two hours
   - C. Three hours
   - D. Five hours

4. Which of the following phases is removed from high copper amalgam alloy?
   - A. Gamma-2 phase
   - B. Alpha-1 phase
   - C. Alpha-2 phase
   - D. Beta phase

5. Which of the followings is/are absent in low copper alloy?
   - A. Zinc
   - B. Palladium
   - C. Indium
   - D. Both B and C

6. High copper alloy should contain at least:
   - A. 6% Cu
   - B. 12% Cu
   - C. 0.01% Cu
   - D. 4% Cu

7. Gamma-1 phase is:
   - A. Ag_3Sn
   - B. Ag_2Hg_3
   - C. $Sn_{7-8}Hg$
   - D. Cu_3Sn

8. Eta phase is:
   - A. Cu_3Sn
   - B. Cu_6Sn_5
   - C. Ag-Cu
   - D. Ag-Sn

9. How much percentage by volume of gamma-1 phase is present in low copper amalgam?
   - A. 20 to 28%
   - B. 30 to 35%
   - C. 54 to 56%
   - D. 65 to 75%

10. Most widely used filling material for posterior teeth is:
   A. Composites
   B. Gold alloy
   C. Amalgam
   D. Zinc oxide-eugenol

11. Percentage of tin in lathe-cut amalgam alloy is:
   A. 63%
   B. 40%
   C. 26%
   D. 15%

12. Which of the following is not a function of silver in amalgam?
   A. Decreases the creep
   B. Increases the strength
   C. Decreases the expansion on setting
   D. Increases tarnish resistance

13. Which of the following acts as scavenger in amalgam alloy?
   A. Silver
   B. Tin
   C. Copper
   D. Zinc

14. Weakest phase of amalgam is:
   A. Ag_3Sn
   B. Ag_2Hg_3
   C. $Sn_{7-8}\,Hg$
   D. Cu-Sn

15. Least stable phase to corrosion in amalgam is:
   A. Gamma-1
   B. Gamma-2
   C. Alpha-1
   D. Epsilon

16. How much copper is present in admixed amalgam alloy powder?
   A. 69%
   B. 27%
   C. 56%
   D. 13%

17. Matrix of admixed type amalgam is formed by:
   A. Gamma-2 phase
   B. Gamma-1 phase
   C. Alpha-1 phase
   D. Eta phase

18. Core of final set single-composition amalgam is formed by:
   A. Ag_3Sn
   B. Ag_2Hg_3
   C. Both of the above
   D. $Sn_{7-8}\,Hg$

19. Self-sealing restorative material is:
   A. Composite
   B. Amalgam
   C. Glass ionomer
   D. Gold alloys

20. Delayed expansion of amalgam is:
   A. 0.01%
   B. 6%
   C. 12%
   D. 4%

21. Delayed expansion usually appears after:
    A. One day   B. Two days
    C. Five days   D. One week

22. Maximum allowable creep of amalgam is:
    A. 0.01%   B. 4%
    C. 3%   D. 0.4%

23. Lowest creep is found in:
    A. Low copper lathe-cut alloy
    B. High copper unicompositional alloy
    C. High copper admixed alloy
    D. Low copper spherical alloy

24. All of the following factors favor contraction *except*:
    A. Low mercury: alloy ratio
    B. Less trituration time
    C. Higher condensation pressure
    D. Smaller particle size

25. Which of the following gases is responsible for delayed expansion of amalgam?
    A. Carbon dioxide   B. Sulfuric oxide
    C. Hydrogen   D. Oxygen

26. Compressive strength of amalgam at one hour generally is:
    A. 60 MPa   B. 80 MPa
    C. 50 MPa   D. 25 MPa

27. What should be the maximum level of nonvolatile residue in mercury?
    A. 0.04%   B. 0.4%
    C. 0.02%   D. 0.2%

28. Hg:alloy ratio for low copper amalgam is:
    A. 1:1   B. 40:60
    C. 60:40   D. 20: 40

29. All of the following are features of over triturated mix *except*:
    A. Decrease in working time
    B. Higher contraction of the amalgam
    C. Strength of lathe-cut alloys is increased, where as it is reduced in high copper alloys
    D. Creep is decreased

30. Size of filler particles in microfilled composite is:
    A. 4-8 μm   B. 8-12 μm
    C. 1-5 μm   D. 0.04-0.4 μm

31. Conventional composite mainly contains:
    A. Ground quartz
    B. Ground silica
    C. Glasses or ceramic containing heavy metals
    D. None of the above

32. Only inorganic filler used in microfilled composite is:
    A. Ceramic containing heavy metals
    B. Colloidal silica
    C. Quartz
    D. None of the above

33. Highest polymerization shrinkage is found in:
    A. Conventional composite
    B. Microfilled composite
    C. Hybrid composite
    D. Small particle composite

34. Best physical and mechanical properties are observed in:
    A. Conventional composite
    B. Small particle composite
    C. Hybrid composite
    D. Microfilled composite

35. Size of filler particles in microfillers is:
    A. 0.10 to 1 μm   B. 0.1 to 100 μm
    C. 0.005 to 0.01 μm   D. 1 to10 μm

36. Polymerization shrinkage in composite resin in:
    A. 0.01 to 0.1%   B. 0.1 to 1.0%
    C. 1.0 to 7.0%   D. 7.0 to 8.9%

37. Filler particle size in a conventional composite is:
    A. 0.04-0.4 μm   B. 8-12 μm
    C. 5-8 μm   D. 1-4 μm

38. Amine accelerator in visible light cure composite is:
    A. Camphoroquinone
    B. Hydroquinone
    C. Benzoyl peroxide
    D. Dimethylaminoethyl-methacrylate

39. **Photoinitiator in visible light cure composite is:**
    A. Hydroquinone
    B. Camphoroquinone
    C. Diethyl-amino-ethyl-methacrylate
    D. Benzoyl peroxide

40. **Highest compressive strength is found in:**
    A. Conventional composite
    B. Hybrid composite
    C. Small particle composite
    D. Microfilled composite

41. **First translucent filling material is:**
    A. Glass ionomer   B. Silicate
    C. Composite   D. Polycarboxylate

42. **The average life of silicate restoration is:**
    A. Eight years   B. Eleven years
    C. Four years   D. Six years

43. **Gold is used principally for the:**
    A. Pit and small class I cavity
    B. Class III and V restorations
    C. Repair of cement vent holes in gold crowns
    D. All of the above

44. **Which of the following types of condenser diameters is mostly used to condense gold?**
    A. 0.1 to 0.5 mm   B. 0.5 to 1.5 mm
    C. 1.5 to 2.0 mm   D. 2.0 to 3.5 mm

45. **Fusion temperature of high fusing compound is:**
    A. Between 1100 and 1300°F
    B. Between 850 and 1100°F
    C. Below 850°F
    D. Above 1300°F

46. **Which of the following methods is/are used to reduce brittleness of porcelain?**
    A. Disruption of crack propagation
    B. Development of residual compressive stresses
    C. Both of the above
    D. None of the above

47. Which of the following methods is/are used to develop residual compressive stresses?
    A. Ion exchange
    B. Thermal tempering
    C. Thermal compatibility
    D. All of the above

48. Which of the following is used in transformation toughening of porcelain?
    A. Cerium oxide
    B. Partially stabilized zirconium
    C. Titanium oxide
    D. Copper oxide

49. Which of the following is not correct about shade matching?
    A. Use of good natural light
    B. Done preferably in morning
    C. Dry the tooth before matching
    D. First basic hue is selected by matching the shade of canine

50. Porcelain is etched by:
    A. Phosphoric acid
    B. Hydrofluoric acid
    C. Ammonium tricholate
    D. Both B and C

51. Maximum part of ceramics is formed by:
    A. Quartz   B. Kaolin
    C. Alumina   D. Feldspar

52. Alumina in ceramics acts as:
    A. Binder   B. Glass former
    C. Filler   D. None of the above

53. How much porcelain shrinks by volume during firing?
    A. 10%   B. 20%
    C. 28%   D. 35%

54. Definite shrinkage is found in:
    A. Low bisque stage
    B. Medium bisque stage
    C. High bisque stage
    D. None of the above

55. **Glazing of porcelain increases its:**
    A. Strength
    B. Esthetics
    C. Hygiene
    D. All of the above

56. **Chemical bonding across the porcelain metal interface is done by:**
    A. Chromium oxide
    B. Titanium oxide
    C. Copper oxide
    D. Both A and B

57. **Which of the following has highest strength among dental porcelains?**
    A. Castable glass ceramics
    B. Magnesia core porcelains
    C. Glass infiltrated alumina core
    D. Glass infiltrated spinel core

58. **IPS Empress is:**
    A. Magnesia core porcelain
    B. CAD-CAM ceramics for inlays
    C. CAD-CAM ceramics for cores
    D. Injection moulded ceramics

59. **DICOR is:**
    A. Leucite- reinforced porcelain
    B. Glass infiltrated spinal core
    C. Castable glass ceramic
    D. Magnesia core porcelain

Answers

1.A. Creep values at amalgam—
    Low copper   2%
    Admixed   0.4%
    Single composition 0.13%

2.D. This delayed expansion sets in after 2-5 days.

3.D. The satisfactory strength of amalgam to bear masticatory forces is around 310 MPa.

4.A. Gamma-2 phase is present though to a lesser extent than in low copper alloys, hence, high copper allays are more resistant to corrosion.

5.D. Palladium and indium are compositions of single composition alloys.

6.A. Two different types of high copper alloy powder are available. The first is an admixed alloy powder and the second is a single-composition alloy powder. Both types contain more than 6 wt% copper.

7.B. $Ag_2 Hg_3$ phase is stable in the oral environment due to lack of tin though dental gamma-1 phase does contain small amount of tin.

8.B. Eta phase (η) is $Cu_6 Sn_5$ and is formed mainly in admixed alloys, and some single composition alloys. γ_2 phase is replaced by η phase.

9.C. The weakest component is the γ phase. The hardness of γ_2 is approximately 10% of the hardness of γ_1, whereas the γ phase hardness is somewhat higher than that of γ_1.

10.C. Amalgam is the material of choice for posterior restorations due to its superior mechanical properties and longevity.

11.C. If the tin concentration exceeds 26.8 wt%, a mixture of γ phase and a thin-rich phase is formed, which increases the amount of tin-mercury phase when the alloy is amalgamated. The tin-mercury phase lacks corrosion resistance and is the weakest component of the dental amalgam.

12.C. ADA specification No.1 requires that amalgam neither contract nor expand more than 20 μm/cm, measured at 37 $^\circ$C, between 5 minutes and 24 hours after the beginning of trituration, with a device that is accurate to at least 0.5 μm.

13.D. Zinc in amalgam alloy acts as a deoxidizer, a scavenger during melting, uniting with oxygen to minimize formation of other oxides.

14.C. This is the gamma-2 phase, which is least stable in the oral cavity and most prone to tarnish and corrosion.

15.B. Refer to Answer No.14

16.D. The total copper content in admixed amalgam alloy powder is 9 wt% to 20 wt%.

17.B. Present in this matrix of gamma-1 phase is an eta phase (Cu_6 Sn_5) and unconsumed alloy of both types of particles.

18.B. Core of final set single composition amalgam is formed by gamma-1 phase.

19.B. The formation of corrosion products at cavity restoration margins over time accounts for the self-sealing property of amalgam restorations.

20.D. 4% expansion indicates 400 µm expansion.

21.C. Most amalgams exhibit little further dimensional change after 24 hours. Delayed expansion usually starts after 3 to 5 days and may continues for months, reaching values greater than 400 µm (4%).

22.C. Maximum allowable creep rate is 3% according to ADA specification No.1.

23.B. The higher the creep, the greater the degree of marginal deterioration (breakdown) of traditional low copper amalgam are severely ditched. However, for low copper amalgams, creep is not necessarily a good predictor of marginal fracture. Many of these amalgams have creep rates of 0.4%.

24.B. Following are several causes for excessive expansion at amalgam:

- Insufficient trituration
- Insufficient condensation
- Delayed expansion.

  Under trituration results in reduced strength and possibly further expansion during hardening.

25.C. Reaction of zinc in amalgam alloy with water present due to moisture contamination leads the formation of hydrogen gas, which accumulates within the restoration and is the cause of delayed expansion in amalgam alloy restorations.

26.B. As stipulated by ADA specification No.1, the one-hour compressive strength of amalgam is 80 MPa.

27.C. As stipulated by United States Pharmacopeia.

28.A. The most obvious method for reducing the Hg content of the restoration is to reduce the original mercury: alloy ratio. This method is known as the minimal mercury technique or the Eames technique. The recommended mercury: alloy ratios for most modern late cut alloys is 1:1 or 50% mercury. With spherical alloys the recommended amount of Hg is close to 42%.

29.D. Undertriturated mix is weak and susceptible to tarnish. Undertrituration or overatrituration decreases the strength for both traditional and high-copper amalgams. Manipulative procedures favoring consumption of mercury and contraction of amalgam are:

  A. Lower mercury: alloy ratios
  B. Higher condensation pressures
  C. Longer triturcation time
  D. Smaller partied size alloys.

30.D. Filler particle size values in composites (μm):

  • Traditional composite   8-12
  • Small particle filled composite 1-5
  • Microfilled composite   0.04-0.4
  • Hybrid composite   0.6-1.0

31.A. Average size of filter particles in conventional composites is 8 to 12 μm. Filler loading for macrofilled generally is 70 to 80 wt% or 60 to 65 vol%.

32.B. This is used in an effort to overcome the problems of surface roughening associated with traditional composites.

33.B. This increased polymerization shrinkage is present due to the incorporation of prepolymensed composite highly loaded with colloidal silica particles to increase filler loading

34.B. To achieve the best physical and mechanical properties, the small particle composites are loaded with inorganic fillers ground to a size smaller than those used in traditional composites.

35.B. Filler particles are mostly produced by grinding or milling quartz or glasses to produce particles ranging in size from 0.1 to 100 μm.

36.C. Most composites only can be practically cured to levels of 50% to 65% degree of conversion of the reactive monomer sites. Polymerization shrinkage for conventional composites is approximately 2 vol%.

37.B. Refer to Answer No. 30

38.D. The amine accelerator is added in a concentration of about 0.15 wt%.

39.B. Camphoroquinone has an absorption range between 400 nm and 500 nm that is the blue region of visible light.

40.C. Compressive strength of various composites is as follows:

Small particle	350-400 MPa
Hybrid	300-350 MPa
Traditional	250-300 MPa
Microfilled	250-350 MPa

41.B. Silicate cement was the first tooth colored restorative material.

42.C. Silicate cement was introduced in 1878 by Fletcher in England. It was recommended for small restorations in the anterior teeth of the patients with high caries activity.

43.D. Restorations made from direct filling gold cannot bear excessive masticatory stresses; therefore, they are used in areas where they merely fill a space.

44.B. Smaller condenser tips are used where less force is desired to be applied.

45.D. High fusing impression compounds or tray compounds are used for making the special trays for corrective wash or final impressions.

46.C. The principal deficiencies of porcelain are:
A. Brittleness
B. Low fracture toughness
C. Low tensile strength.

47.D. Propagation of cracks from surface flaws is responsible for the poor mechanical behavior of ceramics in tension. Flaws within the interior of the material can also caused fracture initiation under certain conditions.

48.B. This technique is a method for strengthening glass by incorporating a crystalline material that is capable of undergoing a change in crystalline structure when placed under stresses.

49.C. Before shade matching, the tooth is generally wet with saliva so as to give the natural look.

50.B. Acidulated phosphate fluoride (APF) is known to etch glass, probably by selective leaching of sodium ions.

51.D. Feldspar can be either potash or sodium feldspar.

52.B. Alumina takes part in the formation of the glass network and it alters softening point and viscosity.

53.D. The purpose of firing is simply to sinter the particles of powder together properly to form the restoration.

54.B. In medium bisque stage, complete cohesion of particles takes place therefore, definite shrinkage occurs in this stage.

55.D. Glazing of porcelain: (a) gives it a highly polished and smoothest surface (b) eliminates all flaws from the surface.

56.A. Fused porcelain diffuses into the metallic oxide layer formed on the surface of the metal and the metallic oxide layer diffuses into porcelain. Therefore it is a combination of chemical and mechanical bonding.

57.B. They can be used with veneer porcelain, which is bonded to metal.

58.D. They are used to form the core layer of all porcelain crowns.

59.C. It consists of hydroxyapatite crystals in a glass matrix.

1. Fineness of eighteen carat gold is:
   A. 750
   B. 1000
   C. 250
   D. 180

2. How much gold is present in type III gold alloy?
   A. 80-85%
   B. 70-80%
   C. 45-50%
   D. 13-17%

3. Highest percentage of copper is found in:
   A. Type III gold alloy
   B. Type I gold alloy
   C. Type IV gold alloy
   D. Type III gold alloy

4. Which of the following types of gold alloy is/are used in short span bridges?
   A. Type III gold alloy
   B. Type IV gold alloy
   C. Type I gold alloy
   D. Type II gold alloy

5. Type IV gold alloy is used for:
   A. Small inlay
   B. Large inlay
   C. Short span bridge
   D. Long span bridge

6. Density of gold is:
   A. $10.4 \, gm/cm^3$
   B. $19.3 \, gm/cm^3$
   C. $14.4 \, gm/cm^3$
   D. $12.4 \, gm/cm^3$

7. Which of the followings has lowest coefficient of thermal expansion?
   A. Gold
   B. Palladium
   C. Silver
   D. Platinum

8. Which of the following base metal alloys is used for removable partial denture?
   A. Cobalt- chromium
   B. Nickel-chromium
   C. Cobalt-chromium-nickel
   D. All of the above

9. Which of the following gold alloys is used as removable partial denture alloys?
   A. Type II gold alloys   B. Type III gold alloys
   C. Both of the above   D. Type IV gold alloys

10. Platinum is present in:
    A. Type II gold alloys   B. Type I gold alloys
    C. Type III gold alloys   D. Type IV gold alloys

11. What should be the maximum content of copper in gold alloys?
    A. 8%   B. 9%
    C. 16%   D. 14%

12. Which of the following elements of gold alloy reduces the grain size?
    A. Platinum   B. Palladium
    C. Silver   D. Copper

13. Which of the followings is added in gold alloys to compensate for coefficient of thermal expansion?
    A. Zinc   B. Indium
    C. Calcium   D. Platinum

14. Casting shrinkage of gold alloys ranges from:
    A. 0.1% to 1.0%   B. 1.0 to 1.25%
    C. 1.25 to 1.65%   D. 1.65 to 2.15%

15. Which of the followings is not correct about hardening heat treatment?
    A. Increases proportional limit
    B. Decreases ductility
    C. Increases hardness
    D. None of the above

16. Which of the followings help in age hardening process?
    A. Silver   B. Copper
    C. Platinum   D. Palladium

17. Which of the followings is/are reduced in solution heat treatment?
    A. Ductility
    B. Strength
    C. Both of the above
    D. None of the above

18. Gold content in economy gold should be below:
    A. 40%   B. 80%
    C. 60%   D. 45%

19. How much palladium should be present in silver palladium alloys?
    A. 20%   B. 60%
    C. 25%   D. 45%

Answers

1.A. Fineness is number of parts of gold per 1000 of gold. 18 karat gold is 75% gold and 25% other metals, therefore, has a fineness of 750.

2.C. According to ADA specification No.5 type III (hard) alloys are used for high stress situations including onlays, crowns, thick veneer crowns and short-span fixed partial dentures.

3.C. Type IV gold alloys have about 14% copper.

4.A. Type I gold alloys—Soft
    Type II gold alloys—Medium
    Type III gold alloys—Hard
    Type IV gold alloys—Extra hard.

5.D. According to ADA specification No.5, type IV (extra hard) alloys are used for extremely high-stress states, such as endodontic posts and cores, thin veneer crowns, long-span fixed partial dentures and removable partial dentures.

6.B. Density of type I gold alloy is highest and decreases as the nobility decreases from type I to metal ceramic alloys. Density of some elements is as follows:
    Iridium-22.5 g/cm^3-highest density
    Platinum-21-45 g/cm^3
    Gold-19.32 g/cm^3
    Tungsten-19.3 g/cm^3

7.D. The coefficient of thermal expansion (CTE) tends to have a reciprocal relationship with the melting point of alloys and the melting range of the alloys, that is, the higher the malting temperature of a metal, the lower its CTE.

8.D. More commonly used alloys are nickel-chromium and nickel-cobalt -chromium.

9.D. Also used for long span bridges and full crowns.

10.D. Platinum, palladium and copper all are effective in reducing the casting shrinkage of an alloy. Platinum content ranges from 3-6 wt%.

11.C. Gold alloys can be significantly hardened if the alloy contains a sufficient amount at copper. Copper also reduces the casting shrinkage.

12.A. In metal ceramic gold alloy porcelain discoloration due to copper is possible but does not appear to be a major problem.

13.D. It was found that adding both platinum and palladium to gold alloys would lower the coefficient of thermal contraction.

14.C. Platinum, palladium and copper all are effective in reducing the casting shrinkage of an alloy.

15.D. All the above changes caused by hardening heat treatment are controlled by the amount of solid state transformations allowed, which in turn are controlled by the temperature and time of age hardening treatment.

16.B. For age hardening of type III gold alloys, copper content should be at least 8 wt%. Age hardening is soaking or aging the casting at a specific temperature (200° C- 400° C) for a definite time (usually 15-30 minutes) before it is water quenched.

17.B. During heating the alloy at 700°C and then rapidly quenching in water, a disordered solid solution is formed and the rapid quenching prevents ordering from occurring during cooling, therefore, strength is reduced.

18.C. Below 60% gold content:
   A. Reduces cost
   B. Provides sufficient good properties of gold
   C. Provides sufficient strength and hardness for long span bridges.

19.C. These alloys are white and predominantly silver in composition but have substantial amounts of palladium (at least 25%) that provide nobility and promote the silver tarnish resistance.

Wrought Base Metal Alloys

1. **How much carbon should be present in carbon steel?**
   A. More than 1.25 weight percent
   B. Less than 1.25 weight percent
   C. More than 0.25 weight percent
   D. Less than 0.25 weight percent

2. **Passivating effect of which of the followings makes steel resistant to tarnish and corrosion?**
   A. Cadmium
   B. Chromium
   C. Zinc
   D. Potassium

3. **Which of the followings is formed due to passivating effect of chromium?**
   A. CrO
   B. $CrCl_3$
   C. Cr_2O_3
   D. $Cr_2(SO_4)_3$

4. **How much carbon is present in chromium steel?**
   A. Less than 0.1 weight percent
   B. Less than 0.2 weight percent
   C. Less than 0.3 weight percent
   D. Less than 0.4 weight percent

5. **Upper limit of carbon in austenitic steel is:**
   A. 1.20% by weight
   B. 0.3% by weight
   C. 2.1% by weight
   D. 0.08% by weight

6. **Nickle is absent in:**
   A. Ferritic steel
   B. Martensitic steel
   C. Austenitic steel
   D. All of the above

7. **How much chromium is present in 18:8 stainless steel?**
   A. 8 weight percent
   B. 18 weight percent
   C. 0.25 weight percent
   D. 74 weight percent

8. **In soldering, liquidus temperature of filler metal should be:**
   A. Above 450°F
   B. Below 450°F
   C. Above 450°C
   D. Below 450°C

9. 18:8 stainless steel when heated between 400°C and 900°C loses its corrosion resistance property due to precipitation of:
   A. Ferrous carbide
   B. Nickel carbide
   C. Chromium carbide
   D. None of the above

10. Number of 90° cold bends without fracture is maximum in orthodontic wire made up of:
    A. Stainless steel
    B. Cobalt-chromium-nickel
    C. Nickel-titanium
    D. β-titanium

11. Which of the following wire alloys has maximum ultimate tensile strength?
    A. Stainless steel
    B. Cobalt-chromium-nickel
    C. Nickel-titanium
    D. β-titanium

12. The soldering temperature of silver solders for stainless steel is:
    A. 450°C- 460°C
    B. 480°C- 490°C
    C. 620°C-665°C
    D. 680°C-710°C

13. Which of the followings is added in soldering flux to dissolve the chromium oxidizing passivating film so that solder can wet the stainless steel?
    A. Sodium fluoride
    B. Potassium fluoride
    C. Borax
    D. Sodium succinate

14. Shape memory phenomenon is found in:
    A. Elgiloy
    B. Nitinol
    C. β-titanium
    D. None of the above

15. Nitinol wires have:
    A. Shape memory phenomenon
    B. Superelasticity
    C. Both of the above
    D. None of the above

16. Superelasticity phenomenon is found in which stage of nitinol wire?
    A. Austenite stage
    B. Martensite stage
    C. Ferrite stage
    D. All of the above

17. Which of the following wires can not be soldered?
    A. β–titanium
    B. Nitinol
    C. Both of the above
    D. None of the above

18. **Total percentage of cobalt, chromium and nickel in cobalt-chromium alloys should not be:**
    A. Less than 95%   B. Less than 80%
    C. Less than 75%   D. Less than 90%

19. **Liquidus temperature of filler metal in brazing should be above:**
    A. 350°C   B. 450°F
    C. 450°C   D. 350°F

20. **Highest modulus of elasticity is found in:**
    A. β-titanium wire
    B. Nickel-titanium wire
    C. Cobalt-chromium-nickel wire
    D. Stainless steel

21. **Percentage by weight of nickel in 18:8 stainless steel is:**
    A. 18%   B. 8%
    C. 2.5%   D. 76%

Answers

1.B. Carbon steels are iron based alloys which usually contain less than 1.2 weight percent carbon.

Carbon steels	Maximum carbon solubility
Ferrite	0.02%
Austenite	2.1%

2.B. Refer to Answer No. 3.

3.C. The passivating effect of chromium is due to the formation of an imperious, thin, transparent but tough layer of chromium oxide, Cr_2O_3, on the surface of the alloy when it is exposed to an oxidizing atmosphere.

4.C. The 18 to 8 stainless steel may lose its resistance to corrosion if it is heated between 400°C and 900°C because of the precipitation of chromium carbide (Cr_3C) at the grain boundaries.

5.C. The austenitic stainless steel alloys are the most corrosion resistant of the stainless steels.

6.A. Composition of ferritic stainless steel:

Chromium	11.5 to 27%
Carbon	0.20%(max.)
Phosphorous	Traces
Sulfur	Traces
Silicon	Traces
Manganese	Traces
Iron	Balance

7.B. Nickel is 8 wt. percent.

8.D. A rule of the thumb is that the liquidus temperature of the filler material should be 100°F (56°C), below the solidus temperature of the substrate material (metal).

9.C. This precipitation of chromium carbide occurs at the grain boundaries at high temperatures.

10.B. A phase change as well as stress relief is probably responsible. Also the modulus of elasticity of cobalt chromium-nickel wires is more than stainless steel wires.

11.A. The value of tensile strength for 18 : 8 stainless steel is 2117 MPa.

12.C. Silver solders are essentially alloys of silver, copper and zinc to which elements such as tin and indium may be added to lower fusion temperatures and improve solderability.

13.B. The soldering material (solder) does not wet the metal when such a film is present.

14.B. Austenite to martensite phase transition results in shape memory and super elasticity (pseudoelasticity).

15.C. Both these properties of nitinol are present due to the phase transition that occurs from austenite to martensite on cooling or on stress application.

16.B. The cobalt content is used to control the lower transition temperature, which can be near mouth temperature (37°C).

17.B. These wires have to be joined by mechanical crimps because they cannot be soldered or welded.

18.C. Wires made from this alloy should not be annealed, because the resulting softening effect cannot be reversed by subsequent heat treatment.

19.C. In soldering, filler metal have a liquidus temperature not exceeding 450°C.

20.C. Modulus of elasticity values (GPa)

Stainless steel	179
Cobalt-chromium-nickel	184
Nickel-titanium	41.4
β titanium	71.7

21.B. Austenitic stainless steel has greater ductility and ability to undergo more cold work without fracturing than any other types.

15   *Dental Investments*

1. **Gypsum bonded investment are used for the casting of:**
   - A. Base metal alloys
   - B. Gold alloys
   - B. Both of the above
   - C. None of the above

2. **Type of expansion in type I investment is:**
   - A. Mainly thermal
   - B. Mainly hygroscopic
   - C. Thermal as well as hygroscopic
   - D. None of the above

3. **Which of the following is/are modifier(s) in investment materials?**
   - A. Tridymite
   - B. Calcium sulfate
   - C. Both of the above
   - D. Sodium chloride

4. **All of the following are present in gypsum bonded investment *except*:**
   - A. Calcium sulfate
   - B. Silica
   - C. Modifiers
   - D. None of the above

5. **Which of the following is/are added in gypsum bonded investment to compensate its shrinkage on heating?**
   - A. Gypsum
   - B. Silica
   - C. Modifiers
   - D. Both B and C

6. **Presence of carbon in investment does not allow the investment to be heated above:**
   - A. 450°C
   - B. 450°F
   - C. 650°C
   - D. 550°C

7. **How much expansion is desired to be present for type II investment?**
   - A. 0.1 to 0.2 %
   - B. 1.0 to 1.2%
   - C. 1.1 to 2.2 %
   - D. 1.3 to 3.3 %

8. Which of the following is/are able to increase the hygroscopic expansion of gypsum bonded investment?
    A. Silica
    B. Finer particles of silica
    C. Alpha hemihydrate gypsum binder
    D. All of the above

9. All of the following affect the hygroscopic expansion of gypsum bonded investment *except*:
    A. Restraining effects of wax patterns
    B. Amount of water present in the wet asbestos lining of the ring
    C. The nature of the asbestos liner
    D. None of the above

10. Highest thermal expansion is found in:
    A. Quartz   B. Cristobalite
    C. Tridymite   D. Fused quartz

11. Thermal expansion of type I investment at 500°C is:
    A. 0.1 to 0.6 %   B. 1.0 to 1.6%
    C. 0.01 to0.06%   D. 1.1 to 2.6%

12. Phosphate bonded investment is used for casting of:
    A. High temperature melting alloys
    B. Metal ceramic restorations
    C. Both of the above
    D. Gold alloys

13. How much silica is present in phosphate bonded investment?
    A. 60%   B. 70%
    C. 75%   D. 80%

14. Which of the following investment materials is used for casting of high-fusing base metal partial denture alloys?
    A. Gypsum bonded
    B. Phosphate bonded
    C. Ethyl silicate bonded
    D. None of the above

15. Which of the following is not an allotropic form of silica?
    A. Quartz   B. Cristobalite
    C. Tridymite   D. None of the above

16. **How much dental stone is present in gypsum bonded investment?**
    A. 60%   B. 65%
    C. 30%   D. 5%

17. **Silica in gypsum bonded investment acts as:**
    A. Refractory during heating the investment
    B. Thermal expansion regulator
    C. Both of the above
    D. None of the above

18. **Setting time of gypsum bonded investment should:**
    A. Not be less than 5 minutes
    B. Less than 90 minutes
    C. Not more than 25 minutes
    D. Both A and C

19. **Which of the following is absent in phosphate bonded investment?**
    A. $NH_4H_2PO_4$
    B. Silica
    C. Magnesium oxide
    D. None of the above

Answers

1.B. According to American Dental Association specification No.2.

2.A. Type I investment   :   Thermal expansion

Type II investment   :   Hygroscopic expansion

3.D. Boric acid and sodium chloride are used as modifying agents to regulate setting expansion and setting time and to prevent shrinkage of gypsum when it is heated above 300°C.

4.D. The α-hemihydrates form of gypsum is generally the binder. Silica is added to provide refractory and to regulate the thermal expansion.

5.D. Silica in investment causes it to expand thermally to compensate partially or totally for casting shrinkage.

6.C. A slight expansion occurs between 400°C and approximately 700°C and then a large contraction occurs due to decomposition and emitted sulfur gases such as sulfur dioxide, which contaminates the castings with the sulfides of silver and copper.

7.C. Minimum setting expansion in water is required to be 1.2% and maximum expansion permitted is 2.2%.

8.D. Hygroscopic setting expansion may be six or more times the normal setting expansion of a dental investment.

9.D. Any water–insoluble powder that is wettable can be mixed with the gypsum hemihydrate, and hygroscopic expansion results.

10.B. When silica is heated, a change in crystalline form (from α or low to β or high form) occurs at a transition temperature characteristic at the particular from of silica.

11.B. According to American Dental Association specification No. 2.

12.C. The definite advantage of this type of investment is that there is less chance for the contamination of the gold alloys during casting.

13.D. This silica can be either in the form of crystobalite or quartz or a mixture of the two.

14.C. In this investment, the binder is silica gel that reverts to silica (cristobalite) on heating

15.D. Quartz, cristobalite or a combination of the two forms may be used in a dental investment.

16.C. The strength of the investment is dependent on the amount of the binder (α-hemihydrate) present. The gypsum-bonded investment may contain 25% to 45% of the gypsum product.

17.C. When the silica is heated at transitional temperature, the density decreases, as the α–form changes to the β form, with a resulting increase in volume that is exhibited by a rapid increase in the linear expansion.

18.D. According to ADA specification No.2, the setting time of gypsum bonded investments should be 5 to 25 minutes. Modern inlay investments set initially in 9 to 18 minutes.

19.D. Ammonium diacid phosphate ($NH_4H_2 PO_4$): It is a ceramic substance, which hardens at room temperature and is responsible for high temperature strength. Silica: Present in the form of quartz or crystobalite produces phosphate ions in solution. Magnesium oxide: Acts as a binder.

16   *Casting Procedure*

1. **Most commonly used die material is:**
   A. Type III dental stone
   B. Type IV dental stone
   C. Electroformed silver die
   D. Silica-filled epoxy resin

2. **Least occlusal dimensional change is found in dies made up of:**
   A. Type IV stone + gypsum hardener A
   B. Type IV stone + gypsum hardener B
   C. Type IV stone
   D. Silica- filled epoxy resin

3. **Thickness of die-spacer should not be more than:**
   A. 0.1 mm   B. 0.2 mm
   C. 0.4 mm   D. 0.5 mm

4. **What should be the direct current level if silver cyanide is used to make electroformed dies?**
   A. 0.1 milli ampere per cm^2 of cathode surface
   B. 1.0 milli ampere per cm^2 of cathode surface
   C. 5.0 milli ampere per cm^2 of cathode surface
   D. None of the above

5. **Sprue former should be attached to which of the following areas of pattern?**
   A. Largest cross-sectional area
   B. Smallest cross-sectional area
   C. Any one of the above
   D. None of the above

6. **Type of porosity caused by hot-spot is:**
   A. Microporosity
   B. Subsurface porosity
   C. Suck- back porosity
   D. Pinhole porosity

7. What should be the level of the top of the wax pattern in relation to the open end of the ring for phosphate bonded investment?
   A. 6.5 mm
   B. 4.5 mm
   C. 3.25 mm
   D. 2.5 mm

8. Thickness of the casting ring liner should be:
   A. 0.5 mm
   B. 0.7 mm
   C. 1.0 mm
   D. 1.5 mm

9. Which of the following is/are used as casting ring liner?
   A. Aluminium silicate ceramic material
   B. Cellulose
   C. Ceramic-cellulose combination
   D. All of the above

10. Maximum prescribed temperature for gypsum bonded investment in hygroscopic expansion technique is:
    A. 650°C
    B. 468°C
    C. 550°C
    D. 450°C

11. Which of the following contaminates gold alloy if gypsum bonded investment is heated above 700°C?
    A. Oxide
    B. Sulfur dioxide
    C. Peroxide
    D. None of the above

12. Which of the following flame zones should be kept away from the metal during fusion?
    A. Mixing zone
    B. Combustion zone
    C. Reducing zone
    D. Oxidizing zone

13. Hottest zone of flame is:
    A. Oxidizing zone
    B. Reducing zone
    C. Combustion zone
    D. Mixing zone

14. Best pickling solution for gypsum bonded investment is:
    A. 50% H_2SO_4
    B. 50% HCl
    C. 50% H_3PO_4
    D. 60% HNO_3

15. A non-carbon investment should be used for casting of:
    A. Ag-Pd alloy
    B. High Pd alloy
    C. Pd-Ag alloy
    D. All of the above

16. Minute ridges or veins on the surface of casting are formed due to:
   A. Air
   B. Water films
   C. Too rapid heating
   D. Too slow heating

17. What should be the range of pressure in an air pressure casting machine?
   A. 0.1 to 0.14 MPa
   B. 15 to 20 psi
   C. Both of the above
   D. None of the above

18. How many turns are sufficient in an average type of centrifugal casting machine for casting of a full coverage molar crown?
   A. One to two turns
   B. Two to three turns
   C. Two to five turns
   D. Four to five turns

19. Increased sprue length increases:
   A. Localized shrinkage porosity
   B. Subsurface porosity
   C. Microporosity
   D. None of the above

20. Black casting occurs due to:
   A. Overheating of investment
   B. Incomplete elimination of wax
   C. Both of the above
   D. None of the above

21. Outermost zone of flame is:
   A. Combustion zone
   B. Reducing zone
   C. Oxidizing zone
   D. Mixing zone

Answers

1.B. Type IV gypsum product, according to ADA specification No.25, is high strength dental stone. Principal requisites for a die material are strength hardness and minimum setting expansion.

2.C. Values of occlsual dimensional change:

Type IV stone	0.06%
Type IV stone + gypsum hardener A	0.16%
Type IV stone + gypsum hardener B	0.10%
Silica filled epoxy resin	0.15%
Aluminum filled epoxy resin	0.14%
Electroformed silver die	0.10%

3.D. Spacers include model paint, colored nail polish or thermoplastic polymers dissolved in volatile solvents. This provides relief for the luting cement and less than 0.5 mm is used to ensure complete seating of an otherwise precisely fitting casting.

4.C. The value of direct current is 5-10 milli ampere per square centimeter of cathode surface for 10 hours.

5.A. It is best for the molten alloy to flow from the largest cross-sectional area to the margins to reduce the risk of turbulence.

6.C. A hot spot is a localized pool of molten metal while the surrounding areas have solidified. This creates a shrinkage void or a suck back type of porosity.

7.C. This length is kept between 3 and 4 mm for the phosphate-bonded investments.

8.C. Most commonly used technique to provide investment expansion is to line walls of the ring with a ring liner.

9.D. Traditionally, asbestos was the material of choice, but it is no longer used because of its carcinogenic potential makes it a biohazard.

10.B. For thermal expansion technique, the maximum temperature can be 650°C.

11.B. The presence of sulfur dioxide in gold castings makes them extremely brittle

$$CaSO_4 + 4C \longrightarrow CaS + 4CO$$
$$3 CaSO_4 + CaS \longrightarrow 4SO_2 + 4CaO.$$

12.D. The temperature of the oxidizing zone is less than that of the reducing zone and it also oxidizes the metal.

13.B. The reducing zone is dimly blue and just lies beyond the green combustion zone. This should always be in contact with the melting metal.

14.B. Hydrochloric acid helps in the removal of residual gypsum bonded investment and also the oxide coating.

15.D. Other alloys that should be invested in a non-carbon investment include nickel-chromium-beryllium, nickel-chromium and cobalt-chromium alloys.

16.B. Too rapid heating rate may cause cracking at the investment, which produces a casting with fins or spines. Small nodules on a casting are caused by air bubbles. Under heating may cause voids or porosity in the castings.

17.C. The pressure-gradient in the centrifugal casting machine is about 0.21 to 0.28 MPa (30 to 40 Psi).

18.C. As the metal fills the mold there is a hydrostatic pressure gradient develops along the length of the casting. The pressure gradient from the tip of the casting to the bottom surface is quite sharp and parabolic in form, reaching zero at the button surface. Solidification progresses from the thin margin edge to the button surface.

19.A. Localized shrinkage porosity results from incomplete feeding of molten metal during solidification. Therefore, if length of sprue is increased, metal will solidify before reaching the casting mould.

20.C. Surface discoloration and roughness can result from sulfur contamination, either from investment breakdown at elevated temperatures or from a high sulfur content of the torch flame. The interaction of the molten alloy with sulfur produces black castings that are brittle and do not clean readily during pickling.

21.C. Refer to Answer No.12.

17 Miscellaneous

1. The process during which a portion of the metal being joined is melted and flowed together is known as:
   A. Soldering
   B. Welding
   C. Brazing
   D. None of the above

2. All of the followings are a type of flux *except*:
   A. Protective
   B. Reducing
   C. Solvent
   D. None of the above

3. The type of flux used to cover the metal surface and prevent access to oxygen so that no oxide can form is:
   A. Reducing flux
   B. Solvent flux
   C. Protective flux
   D. None of the above

4. Which of the following types of fluxe/s is/are used with noble metal alloys?
   A. Boric acid
   B. Boric anhydride
   C. Borax
   D. All of the above

5. Fluoride fluxes are used to dissolve:
   A. Chromium oxide
   B. Cobalt oxide
   C. Nickel oxide
   D. All of the above

6. Compatibility of brazing filler metal consists of:
   A. Appropriate flow temperature
   B. Ability to wet the parent metal
   C. Sufficient fluidity
   D. All of the above

7. By how much the flow temperature should be lower than solidus temperature of the metals being joined?
   A. 150°F
   B. 50°F
   C. 150°C
   D. 56°C

8. Which of the following fuels is associated with highest flame temperature?
   A. Hydrogen
   B. Natural gas
   C. Propane
   D. Acetylene

9. Which of the following fuels is associated with highest heat content?
   A. Acetylene
   B. Propane
   C. Natural gas
   D. Hydrogen

10. Transmission of heat by means of air currents is known as:
    A. Radiant heat
    B. Conduction
    C. Convection
    D. None of the above

11. Passivation effect is shown by:
    A. Chromium
    B. Titanium
    C. Both of the above
    D. None of the above

12. Chemical corrosion is exemplified by:
    A. Halogenation
    B. Reduction
    C. Carbonization
    D. All of the above

13. Which of the following has zero electrode potential?
    A. Gold
    B. Antimony
    C. Hydrogen
    D. Potassium

14. Which of the following has highest positive electrode potential?
    A. Mercury
    B. Potassium
    C. Platinum
    D. Gold

15. What is the approximate value of current when a gold and an amalgam restoration are in the same mouth, but not in contact?
    A. 0.01 to 0.1 milli ampere
    B. 0.5 to 1.0 micro ampere
    C. 0.01 to 0.1 micro ampere
    D. 0.5 to 1.0 milli ampere

16. Crevice corrosion is also known as:
    A. Stress corrosion
    B. Concentration cell corrosion
    C. Galvanic corrosion
    D. None of the above

17. Which of the following does not show passivating effect?
    A. Chromium
    B. Aluminium
    C. Titanium
    D. None of the above

18. Oxidation of alloy particles in dental amalgam is an example of:
    A. Dry corrosion
    B. Galvanic corrosion
    C. Heterogeneous composition corrosion
    D. Concentration cell corrosion

19. Stabilization of stainless steel is done by:
    A. Chromium   B. Titanium
    C. Aluminum   D. Iron

20. For alloy to be protected from corrosion, what should be the minimum percentage of chromium in alloy?
    A. 6%   B. 8%
    C. 10%   D. 12%

21. Base metal alloys use:
    A. Boric acid flux   B. Boric anhydride flux
    C. Both of the above   D. Fluoride flux

22. What should be optimum gap between substrate metal parts to be joined by soldering?
    A. 0.01 to 0.1 mm   B. 0.13 to 0.3 mm
    C. 0.3 to 1.0 mm   D. 0.8 to 1.5 mm

23. Which of the following term include a number of different minerals that possess similar physical properties and crystalline form?
    A. Emery   B. Garnet
    C. Kieselguhr   D. Rouge

24. Rouge is:
    A. Ferric oxide   B. Iron oxide
    C. Chromic oxide   D. Silicon carbide

25. Crocus cloth contains:
    A. Garnet   B. Diatomaceous earth
    C. Rouge   D. Tin oxide

26. Which of the following is used as polishing agent for noble metal alloys?
    A. Tin oxide   B. Chromic oxide
    C. Iron oxide   D. Aluminium oxide

27. All of the followings are desirable properties of an abrasive *except*:
    A. Abrasive should be regular in shape
    B. Abrasive should be harder than the work it abrades
    C. It should possess high impact strength
    D. It should possess attrition resistance

28. Which of the followings has highest Knoop hardness number?
    A. Emery   B. Silicon carbide
    C. Boron carbide D. Diamond

29. Polishing agent for stainless steel is:
    A. Chromic oxide B. Iron oxide
    C. Tin oxide   D. Tripoli

30. Which of the followings is used as polishing agent in dental prophylactic pastes?
    A. Silicon carbide   B. Boron carbide
    C. Zirconium silicate D. Kieselguhr

31. Carrageenan in dentifrices acts as:
    A. Humectant B. Binder
    C. Detergent D. Abrasive

32. Most commonly used implant is:
    A. Endosseous   B. Subperiosteal
    C. Transosteal D. None of the above

33. How much chromium is present in cobalt-chromium-molybdenum-based alloy?
    A. 63% B. 30%
    C. 5%   D. 2%

34. How many times modulus of elasticity of titanium is higher than bone?
    A. Two times   B. Ten times
    C. Twelve times D. Fifteen times

35. Tartar controlling agent in dentifrices is:
    A. Sodium monofluorophosphate
    B. Carrageenan
    C. Disodium pyrophosphate
    D. Potassium nitrate

36. **How much abrasive is present in powder form of dentifrices?**
    A. 65%
    B. 95%
    C. 45%
    D. 25%

37. **Which of the following acts as detergent in dentifrices?**
    A. Diabasic calcium phosphate dihydrate
    B. Sodium lauryl sulfate
    C. Carrageenan
    D. Strontium chloride

38. **Vitallium is composed of:**
    A. Iron-chromium-nickel-based alloy
    B. Titanium-6 aluminium–4 vanadium-based alloy
    C. Cobalt-chromium-molybdenum alloy
    D. Nickel- titanium alloy

39. **Non-bioactive ceramic is:**
    A. Hydroxyapatite
    B. Bioglass
    C. Sapphire
    D. None of the above

40. **Elgiloy is composed of:**
    A. Pd-Ag alloy
    B. Cr-Ni alloy
    C. Co-Cr-Ni alloy
    D. Ni-Ti alloy

41. **Which of the following has highest linear coefficient of thermal expansion?**
    A. Amalgam
    B. Pit and fissure resin
    C. Silicon impression material
    D. Denture resin

42. **The strength of dental investment for gold alloy is dependent on the amount of:**
    A. Silica
    B. Carbon
    C. Copper
    D. Gypsum

43. **Which cement base has the highest elastic modulous:**
    A. Zinc phosphate
    B. Polymer-reinforced ZOE
    C. Zinc polycarboxylate
    D. Glass-ionomer cement

44. **Maximum permissible setting expansion of high strength stone is:**
    A. 0.1%
    B. 0.05%
    C. 0.3%
    D. 0.2%

45. Coefficient of thermal expansion of currently available porcelain is:
    A. 6×10^{-6} /°C
    B. 8×10^{-6}/°C
    C. 10×10^{-6}/°C
    D. 14×10^{-6}/°C

46. The following is the list of elastomeric impression material, which is the most biocompatible?
    A. Polysulfide
    B. Polyether
    C. Addition silicone
    D. Condensation silicone

47. Monophase elastomeric impression materials are based on:
    A. Putty
    B. Heavy body
    C. Regular body
    D. Light body

48. Passivating elements are:
    A. Cr, Al, Ti
    B. Cr, Mo, Ti
    C. Cr, Fe, Mo
    D. Cr, Gold, Ti

49. Crucible indicated for casting base metal alloys is:
    A. Carbon crucible
    B. Clay crucible
    C. Quartz crucible
    D. High melting plastic crucible

50. Which of the following wax coating is present on dental floss?
    A. Beswax
    B. Spermaceti wax
    C. Japan wax
    D. Carnauba wax

51. Which of the following is not a mouth temperature wax:
    A. Adaptol
    B. Korrecta type I
    C. HL physiologic paste
    D. IOWA wax

52. Which of the following dental material shows most tear resistance?
    A. Polysulfide
    B. Condensation silicone
    C. Addition silicone
    D. Polyether

53. Which of the following has the highest modulus of elasticity?
    A. Dentin
    B. Enamel
    C. Amalgam
    D. Composite resin

54. Magnesium oxide is added in zinc phosphate cement to:
    A. Act as an inactive filler
    B. Impart smoothness to freshly mixed cement
    C. Reduce the temperature of calcination process
    D. Lengthen setting time

55. **The Gamma phase in the set dental amalgam refers to:**
    A. Silver-mercury phase   B. Tin-mercury phase
    C. Silver-tin phase   D. Copper-tin phase

Answers

1.B. This can be accomplished either by application of heat or pressure or both, with or without a filler metal.

2.D. Reducing flux: This reduces any oxides present on metal surface and exposes clean metal.

Solvent flux: This dissolves any oxides present and carries them away.

Protective flux: This covers metal surfaces and prevents exposure to oxygen and formation of oxides.

3.C. Refer to Answer No. 2.

4.D. These also act as protective fluxes by forming low temperature glass. These act as reducing fluxes for low stability oxides like copper oxide.

5.D. Fluorides act as solvent fluxes.

6.D. The filler metal should also be color compatible and tarnish and corrosion resistant.

7.D. 56°C or 100°F.

8.D. Acetylene has highest flame temperature (3140° C).

9.B. A lower heat content of fuel is associated with more danger at oxidation during the soldering process.

10.C. Conduction is transmission by conductance through the furnace structure. Radiant heat is transmission by radiation from the heating coils.

11.C. Chromium forms $Cr_2 O_3$ (chromium oxide) on the surface of stainless steel. Besides titanium, aluminum is also a passivating metal.

12.A. Chemical corrosion is due to direct combination of metallic and non-metallic elements. It is exemplified by oxidation, halogenation or sulfurization reactions, that is, discoloration of silver by sulfur.

13.C. Metals with a more positive potential have a lower tendency to dissolve in aqueous environments. The metal with the lowest electrode potential goes into solution.

14.D. Auric (Au 3^+) — + 1.36

Aurous (Au$^+$) — + 1.50

15.B. With this current, the corresponding existing electromotive force (EMF) is 500 mV.

16.B. Crevice corrosion exists whenever there are variations in the electrolytes or in the composition of the given electrolytes within the system.

17.A. Refer to Answer No.11.

18.A. Dry corrosion occurs in the absence of water.

19.B. Stabilization of stainless steel employs successful application of an element that precipitates a carbide in preference to chromium thereby counteracting the decreased corrosion resistance.

Titanium is introduced in an amount 6 times the carbon content.

20.D. The chromium content varies between 12 and 30%.

21.D. Fluoride acts as a solvent flux.

22.B. The optimum gap between parts of substrate metal to be joined has never been defined.

23.B. These minerals are the silicates of aluminum, cobalt, iron, magnesium and manganese.

24.B. Iron oxide is the fine, red abrasive component of rouge. It is used to polish high noble metal alloys.

25.C. Rouge composed of iron oxide. It is an excellent polishing agent for gold and noble metal alloys, but is likely to be dirty to handle.

26.C. Refer to Answer No. 24.

27.A. In dentistry, the outermost particles or surface material of an abrading instrument is referred to as the abrasive.

28.D. Diamond has highest Knoop hardness value (7,000 to 10,000).

29.A. Tin oxide is an extremely fine abrasive used for polishing teeth and metallic restorations in the mouth.

30.C. Zirconium silicate is also known as ZIRCON and is an off-white mineral.

31.B. It prevents solid and liquid separation.

32.A. Various shapes in which endosseous implants are available are blades, screws, hollow cylinders, cones is cylinders with porous surfaces.

33.B. The Co-Cr alloys typically contain—
Cobalt   53–67 wt%
Chromium   25–32 wt%
Molybdenum   2–6 wt%
Chromium has passivating effect and molybdenum is effective hardner and grain refiner.

34.B. Modulus of elasticity of titanium is half that of stainless steel or cobalt-chromium alloys and five to ten times of bone.

35.C. Other tartar controlling agents are—tetrasodium pyrophosphate, tetrapotassium pyrophosphate.

36.B. Varies between 90% and 98%.

37.B. Detergent aids in debris removal.

38.C. Fe-Cr alloy is known as pentilium P-D.

39.C. The same family of non-bioactive ceramics also includes alumina.

40.C. This alloy was originally used for watch springs.

41.C. Dental amalgam–25
Denture resin–81
Pit and fissure resin–85
Elastomeric impression materials–150-220

42.D. Gypsum-bonded investments are used for conventional gold alloys. Most investments now contain α–hemihydrate as a binder, because greater strength is obtained.

43.A. Zinc phosphate has highest elastic modulus.

Zinc phosphate	13.5 GPa
Glass-ionomer	7.3 GPa
Polycarboxylate	5.1 GPa
Polymer-reinforced ZOE	2.5 GPa

44.A. Gypsum product setting expansion at 2 hours:

Type I	0.00-0.15%
Type II	0.00-0.30 %
Type III	0.00-0.20 %
Type IV	0.00-0.10%
Type V	0.10-0.30%

45.D. To bond to alloys suitable for the copings, porcelains must be sufficiently low fusing and they also must have a coefficient of thermal contraction that is closely matched to that of the alloys.

46.A. The set polyether impression material did produce the higher cell toxicity scores and the lowest viable cell count after multiple cell exposures.

47.C. With monophase or a single-viscosity material, only one mix is made and part of the material is placed in the tray and another portion is put in the syringe for injecting into the cavity preparation.

48.D. Formation at a layer of oxide on the surface of these elements prevents tarnish and corrosion. This is called passivating effect. Noble metals resist corrosion because their EMF is positive with regard to any of the common reduction reactions found in the oral environment.

49.C. Carbon crucible for high noble crown and bridge gold alloys and high fusing gold based metal ceramic alloys.

Clay crucible for high noble and noble type alloys.

50.B. Beeswax is insect wax. Spermaceti (animal wax) is obtained from the sperm of whale.

51.A. Working temperature of adoptol wax is not suitable to work in oral cavity temperature.

52.A. Polysulfides have the highest resistance to tearing. However, because of its susceptibility to distortion, it is possible that the polysulfide impressions may distort rather than tear.

53.B. Enamel–4.6 × 10^4 MPa

Dentine–1.4 × 10^4 MPa

Amalgam–3.4 × 10^4 MPa

Composite–resin–1.4 × 10^4 MPa.

54.B. It also aids in sintering

55.C. Gamma phase of dental amalgam is Ag_3Sn.

1. **Torsional force is:**
   A. Compression
   B. Tensile force
   C. Shear
   D. Transverse bending force

2. **Amalgam achieves 70% of the strength by:**
   A. 2 hours
   B. 4 hours
   C. 8 hours
   D. 16 hours

3. **The range of wavelength of visible light curing system is:**
   A. 400-700 nm
   B. 410-500 nm
   C. 365-400 nm
   D. 700-900 nm

Answers

1.C. Shear stress resist the sliding of one portion of a body over another. It is produced by rotational action. It is calculated by dividing the force by the area parallel to the direction of force.

2.C. Generally the strength of amalgam is measured in term of compressive strength. For satisfactory amalgam restoration the compressive strength should be at least 310 MPa. This much force is achieved in about 1 week while the 70% of the strength is achieved in 8 hours.

3.B. Restorative resins polymerize either by chemical activation or by light activation. For light activation visible light is used. It has wavelength of 400 to 500 nanometer.

1. Which of the following statements is true regarding lathe-cut silver alloy?
   A. Requires least amount of mercury
   B. Achieves lowest compressive strength at 1 hour
   C. Has tensile strength, both at 15 minutes and 7 days is comparable to high copper, unicompositional alloys
   D. Has lower creep value

2. Corrosion of amalgam restoration:
   A. Can extend upto a depth of 100 to 500 μm
   B. Decreases if tin content of alloy increases
   C. Is promoted by gamma phase of alloy particles
   D. Is resisted the most by copper–tin phase in high copper amalgams

3. Over-trituration of silver alloy and mercury:
   A. Reduces contraction
   B. Increases the strength of lathe-cut alloy but reduces the strength of spherical alloy amalgam
   C. Decreases creep
   D. Gives a dull and crumbly amalgam mix

4. Which of the following is true about agar hydrocolloid impression material?
   A. Liquefies between 71-100°C
   B. Solidifies between 50-70°C
   C. Facilitates fabrication of metal dyes
   D. Can not register fine surface details

5. Which of the following is not true about elastomeric impression?
   A. Single mix materials have higher viscosity
   B. Shear thinning is related to viscosity of mono phase impression material
   C. Improper mixing of material can cause permanent deformation of impression
   D. Putty-wash technique of impression reduces dimensional change on setting

6. Impression material of choice in patients with submucous fibrosis is:
   A. Zinc oxide-eugenol
   B. Addition silicon
   C. Condensation silicon
   D. Plaster of Paris

7. How soon after contamination by moisture does zinc containing amalgam restoration start expanding?
   A. 12 hours
   B. 1 to 2 days
   C. 3 to 5 days
   D. One week

8. Creep value of which of the following is the highest?
   A. Low copper amalgam alloy
   B. Admix alloy
   C. Single composition alloys
   D. Creep value of all the above-mentioned alloys is same

9. Which of the following cements bonds to tooth structure, which has an anticariogenic effect, has a degree of translucency and does not irritate the pulp?
   A. Polycarboxylate cement
   B. Resin cement
   C. Silicate cement
   D. Glass ionomer cement

10. How much fraction of methyl mercury is absorbed from the gut:
   A. 20%
   B. 50%
   C. 80%
   D. 100%

11. What fraction of inhaled mercury vapor is retained in the body?
   A. 45 to 55%
   B. 55 to 65%
   C. 65 to 85%
   D. >85%

12. The lowest blood mercury level at which the earliest non-specific symptom starts appearing at:
   A. 25 ng/ml
   B. 35 ng/ml
   C. 40 ng/ml
   D. 45 ng/ml

Answers

1.C. The compressive strength of low copper amalgam is low than high copper amalgam while the tensile strength of amalgam is very low of both low copper and high copper amalgam. After 15 minutes both have tensile strength in the range of 4 to 7 MPa and after 24 hours between 48 and 70 MPa. There is no significant increase in tensile strength even after 7 days in case of high copper alloy.

2.D. In high copper alloy either admix or unicomposition type the final phase formed is $Cu_6 Sn_5$. This copper tin phase is less corrosion prone than the Sn-Hg (gamma -2) phase of low copper alloy. However, the copper tin phase is most corrosion prone in the amalgam.

3.B. Both compressive and tensile strength of irregular shaped (lathe-cut) alloy increases by overtrituration. However, compressive and tensile strength of spherical alloys are greatest at normal trituration and on overtrituration decreases. Overtrituration increases creep while undertrituration lowers it.

4.A. The physical change of agar from sol to gel and vice versa is due to temperature change. The gel is heated to 70° to 100°C to return into the sol condition. This temperature is called liquefaction temperature.

5.A. Single mix materials are equivalent to light body single syringe material so they have less viscosity. The excess polymerization shrinkage of condensation silicone recommends for putty-wash technique of impression to have better accuracy and the putty have higher viscosity.

6.B. Submucous fibrosis patient shows limited amount of mouth opening and loss of elasticity of cheek muscles so the impression material used should have less bulk of material and should be elastic. Addition silicon are used for SMF patient as it is most ideally elastic material.

7.C. If zinc-containing amalgam is contaminated by moisture during trituration or condensation large expansion occur. This starts after 3 to 5 days and is known as delayed expansion. This expansion is absent in zinc-free amalgam.

8.A. Creep is time dependent plastic strain of a material under constant load. In amalgam high creep causes greater degree of marginal deterioration. Creep value of low copper amalgam is 0.8% to 8% while high coppers amalgam has creep of even less then 0.1%.

9.A. Anticariogenic effect of cement is due to fluoride release. Fluoride releasing cement is silicate, GIC, silicophosphate and polycarboxylate. Among these least pulp irritation is caused by polycarboxylate cement hence the answer of choice. Glass ionomer cements lacks translucency.

10.D. Methyl mercury is generally formed by biologic action on elemental mercury.

11.C. Inhalation of mercury is at concern in considering the contribution of mercury absorption from dental amalgam.

12.B. The average mercury level in blood of subjects with amalgam fillings was 0.7 ng/ml (coefficient of variation =78%), whereas the level in subjects without amalgam fillings was 0.3 ng/ml (coefficient of variation = 77%).